Lecture Notes:
Medical Law and Ethics

Philip Howard MA (Oxon) MD (Lond) FRCP (Edin) FRCP (Lond)

Consultant physician and Senior Lecturer in medicine
Epson and St Helier University Hospitals NHS Trust
and St George's Hospital Medical School

James Bogle TD BA Dip Law ACIArb

Barrister of the Middle Temple
10 King's Bench Walk
Inner Temple
London

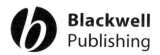
Blackwell
Publishing

Blackwell Publishing, Inc., 350 Main Street, Malden, Massachusetts 02148-5020, USA
Blackwell Publishing Ltd, 9600 Garsington Road, Oxford OX4 2DQ, UK
Blackwell Publishing Asia Pty Ltd, 550 Swanston Street, Carlton, Victoria 3053, Australia

First published 2005

Library of Congress Cataloging-in-Publication Data

Howard, Philip, MD.
    Lecture Notes: Medical Law and Ethics / Philip Howard, James Bogle.
       p. ; cm.
    Includes bibliographical references.
    ISBN 1-4051-1868-7 (alk. paper)
    1. Medical ethics.   2. Medical jurisprudence – Great Britain.
       [DNLM: 1. Jurisprudence – Great Britain.   2. Ethics, Clinical – Great
    Britain.   3. Ethics, Medical – Great Britain.   4. Legislation, Medical –
    Great Britain.   W 32.5 FA1 H851L 2004]   I. Bogle, James.   II. Title.

    R724.H69 2004
    174.2–dc22   2004015946

ISBN 1-4051-1868-7

A catalogue record for this title is available from the British Library

Set in 8/12 Stone Serif by SNP Best-set Typesetter Ltd., Hong Kong
Printed and bound in India by Replika Press Pvt. Ltd.

Commissioning Editor: Vicki Noyes
Development Editor: Geraldine Jeffers
Production Controller: Kate Charman

For further information on Blackwell Publishing, visit our website:
http://www.blackwellpublishing.com

The publisher's policy is to use permanent paper from mills that operate a sustainable forestry policy, and which has
been manufactured from pulp processed using acid-free and elementary chlorine-free practices. Furthermore, the
publisher ensures that the text paper and cover board used have met acceptable environmental accreditation
standards.

Contents

Part 1—Sources of Medical Law and Ethics

1. Nature and origins of medical ethics 3
2. Sources of medical law 16

Part 2—Consent, Confidentiality and Clinical Negligence

3. Consent to treatment 25
4. Confidentiality 39
5. Clinical negligence 47

Part 3—Mental Health

6. Mental health 65
7. Adults with Incapacity (Scotland) Act 2000 79

Part 4—Issues

8. The law in relation to abortion 89
9. The ethics of abortion 99
10. Reproductive technology and surrogacy 109
11. The law in relation to end-of-life issues 116
12. The ethics of end-of-life issues 126
13. Clinical research 137

Part 5—Maintaining Standards and Professional Regulation

14. Maintaining standards and professional regulation 149
15. Presenting evidence and rules of procedure 158
16. The Coroner's court 164
17. The General Medical Council 171

Part 6—Doctors' Rights

18. Employment and other rights of doctors 179

Appendix 1. Philosophers who have influenced medical ethics 184
Appendix 2. Suggested further reading 189
Appendix 3. How to access legal reference materials 193
Appendix 4. Cases 195
Appendix 5. Statutes 199

Index 200

Disclaimer

This book is intended as a general reference guide for medical and nursing students in training or for young health care professionals in practice seeking an introduction to medical law and ethics. It is not intended to be used as a specific reference text for the resolution of particular legal problems. Specific questions regarding any particular issue or any advice about a legal problem should be sought from a qualified legal practitioner. Although every effort has been made to ensure the accuracy of the text, the authors and publisher cannot accept responsibility for any errors or omissions or for any consequences which might occur as a result of such.

Preface

This book is aimed predominantly at medical students. However, we hope that it will also be of practical use for junior doctors in their pre-registration year and in the first few years of clinical practice. The book covers the entire field from everyday matters such as consent to treatment and confidentiality to the more contentious and complex issues such as the moral status of the human embryo in relation to abortion and reproductive technology.

The rising tide of litigation means that no doctor is immune from medico-legal liability for their actions. Clinical negligence claims may threaten the reputation and career of even the most eminent practitioner. No doctor or nurse is free from complaints. There is an increasing public interest in medico-legal matters and concern about the way healthcare professionals are regulated. Public debate has been fuelled by recent scandals such as Shipman, Alder Hey and Bristol and advances in medical science, such as human cloning technology. It is important to understand the organizational changes that have recently come about to deal with complaints and professional accreditation and regulation.

In 1993 the GMC identified medical law and ethics as an important component of the core curriculum. Medical law is fast emerging as an academic discipline within the medical course. As such it requires assessment and is fast becoming an examination subject for Finals, while it already has an established place in the MRCP exam. We have therefore tried to identify the essential or core knowledge, as well as what is practically useful in everyday clinical practice and also what is of interest, or importance, in terms of understanding the subject and the areas of current growth and development. However, we need to recognize that the core curriculum in medical law will be a function of those changes in the law that, in recent times,

have begun to be ever more frequent; and no doctor can afford to ignore such changes.

Our book has three aims.

1 First, to provide a knowledge and understanding of the law in relation to medical practice on a 'need to know basis'. Clearly, not every aspect of medical law will be important to all doctors. Hence, psychiatrists will need a working knowledge of the Mental Health Act, while Gynaecologists will be aware of the Abortion Act but need only rarely consider mental health legislation.

2 Second, to provide practical advice on issues that, while not necessary for examination purposes, may nevertheless be required in practice. Such issues include how to prepare a witness statement or appear before a Coroner's Court.

3 Third, to provide an understanding of the ethical issues that underlie medical law and the contemporary debates and controversies connected with it. The learning objectives to each chapter therefore include:

- Core knowledge—what you need to know.
- Clinical applications—what is of particular relevance in practice.
- Discussion of the background principles and case law.

The learning objectives seek to enable the student:

- To attain a knowledge of medical law as applied to medical practice.
- To develop an understanding of the ethical basis of medical practice.
- To understand the workings of the legal system, the role of the GMC and the Coroner's courts.
- To develop practical skills such as obtaining consent, maintaining confidentiality, writing witness statements, and handling complaints.
- To develop a critical awareness of the major ethico-legal issues, so as to be able to engage in effective communication and dialogue with patients, colleagues, managers and others.

Preface

We are aware that for many students it is only during the pre-registration year that their general
medical education is completed. It is then that
they will put into practice what they have learnt
before qualification. The registration year is an apprenticeship in which the newly qualified doctor
develops through practice the clinical and ethical
skills required of a registered medical practitioner.

The teaching of medical law and ethics should
be 'vertical', and run through the pre-clinical
and clinical curriculum. It should also be
'horizontal', and integrate with the acquisition of
the clinical skills of the particular specialities. We
hope therefore that this book will be of use
throughout medical school and into the early years
of practice.

Dr Philip Howard
Mr James Bogle
August 2004

Part 1

Sources of Medical Law and Ethics

Chapter 1

Nature and origins of medical ethics

Learning objectives

Core knowledge
- Hippocratic tradition
- Ethical systems
- Beliefs of major religions

Clinical applications
- Understanding the ethical perspectives and beliefs of patients and colleagues
- Attitudes regarding respect for the person, death and dying

Background principles
- Religious and secular ethical systems

The purpose of this chapter is to introduce the subject of medical ethics and to emphasize the rich heritage of moral philosophy that has developed since the time of Hippocrates. Medical ethics is the application of moral reasoning to the problems confronting doctors in practice. It is an emerging academic discipline in its own right. An understanding of moral philosophy is as important to medical ethics as a knowledge of physiology is to the practice of clinical medicine. All doctors will be challenged by colleagues and patients on their ethical views in the face of particular dilemmas. Such problems may occur frequently in some areas of practice, such as end-of-life issues on the Intensive Care (ITU) or Neonatal Units or in palliative care.

Many ethical issues in medicine remain contentious and controversial. The stances taken by doctors and patients will reflect their personal, philosophical and religious backgrounds. In a multicultural society it is important to understand religious beliefs and practices. Most hospital Chaplaincies will have some information regarding the views taken by the great world religions about death and dying. It is important for doctors to be aware of these when they are responsible for the care of the dying and their families.

However, it seems unlikely that there will be many examination questions in Finals on the principles of medical ethics *per se*. Nevertheless we hope that this chapter will be of some interest as a general introduction and to those who are interested in Special Study Modules (SSMs) or even in interacted BSc or MA degrees in medical ethics.

The need for medical ethics

No doctor can avoid having to make difficult ethical decisions. While the science of medicine can indicate how a disease should be treated, the decision to treat a particular patient involves other considerations of an ethical nature.

One can explain how to ventilate a patient in ITU. However, this does not answer the question of whether one should ventilate a patient with end-stage chronic airways disease. One may know exactly how to resuscitate a patient, but this knowledge cannot tell a doctor whether he or she should give cardio-pulmonary resuscitation (CPR) to a patient with terminal cancer. An understanding of epilepsy and its treatment will not answer the question whether or not it is right to inform the DVLA about an epileptic who refuses to stop driving and poses a risk to himself or to others on the roads. Microbiological science cannot answer the questions surrounding confidentiality and contact-tracing for those with sexually transmitted disease. What are the limits of confidentiality in the face of a risk of passing on life-threatening HIV infection? While the 'how' of medical practice is a matter of science and technology, the 'why' is a matter of medical ethics (Table 1.1).

What is medical ethics?

The term ethics comes from the Greek word *ethikos*, an adjective meaning 'having to do with character' that is derived from the noun *ethos*, which itself means 'character'. A profession is a group of individuals who are bound by a common ethic or code of conduct.

Ethics can be divided into practical (or applied) ethics and theoretical ethics. Practical ethics concerns the application of ethical standards in practice. Theoretical ethics attempts to understand the underlying basis, assumptions and implications of ethical systems. Most doctors will be con-

cerned mainly with practical ethics. However, some understanding of the underlying basis of medical ethics is useful, just as a knowledge of pathology and pharmacology is important for the practice of medicine.

Medical ethics is concerned with the ethical obligations of doctors to their patients, to their colleagues and to society. In 1999 the European Federation of Internal Medicine, the American Society of Internal Medicine and the American Board of Internal Medicine combined to launch the Medical Professionalism Project, which recently published a document entitled 'Medical professionalism in the new millennium: a Physicians' Charter' (Table 1.2).

The Charter lays down 'three fundamental principles as a set of definitive professional responsibilities'.

- Principle of primacy of patient welfare

  This is based upon a 'dedication to serving the interests of the patient. Altruism contributes to the trust that is central to the physician–patient relationship.'

- Principle of patient autonomy

  'Physicians must have respect for patient autonomy. Physicians must be honest with their patients and empower them to make informed decisions about their treatment. Patients' decisions about their care must be paramount, as long as those decisions are in keeping with

Table 1.1 Why do we need to understand medical ethics?

- Difficult ethical dilemmas are now commonplace.
- Clinical decisions are increasingly questioned by patients, relatives and the courts, e.g. CPR, withdrawal of treatment (especially fluids), ITU care.
- 'How-to-treat' questions are a matter of medical science.
- 'Why-to-treat' issues are a matter of medical ethics.
- Medical ethics is based on moral philosophy.
- There is a rationale behind medical ethics, just as there is behind medical practice.
- Medical ethics is not defined by medical law, except for the 'legal positivist'.
- Not everything that is unethical is illegal—e.g. advertising.

Table 1.2 Professionalism in the new millennium: a Physicians' Charter

'Professionalism is the basis of medicine's contract with society. It demands placing interests of patients above those of the physician, setting and maintaining standards of competence and integrity, and providing expert advice to society in matters of health. Essential to this contract is public trust in physicians, which depends on the integrity of both individual physicians and the whole profession. The medical profession everywhere is embedded in diverse cultures and national traditions, but its members share the role of healer, which has roots extending back to Hippocrates.'

ethical practice and do not lead to demands for inappropriate care.'

- Principle of social justice

'The medical profession must promote justice in the healthcare system, including the fair distribution of healthcare resources. Physicians should work actively to eliminate discrimination in healthcare.'

The Charter also proposes a set of specific professional responsibilities (Table 1.3).

The ethical basis of medical practice

Ethics and reason

In this book it is only possible to give a brief outline of some of the ethical systems which have formed the basis for ethical decision-making. Nevertheless, some conceptual framework is necessary if ethical thinking is to be understood.

To begin our understanding of ethics we might begin with the following assertions:
- Human beings are moral agents and can determine their actions through reflection and choice.
- Justice demands that moral actions are equitable, impartial and principled.
- Moral decisions should treat all equally and be open to rational scrutiny.

Reason must be used to provide an understanding of the basis of ethics and to explain why we ought to act ethically. Moral debate is itself an appeal to

Table 1.3 Professional responsibilities of doctors

- Professional competence
- Honesty with patients
- Patient confidentiality
- Maintaining appropriate relations with patients
- Improving quality of care
- Improving access to care
- Just distribution of finite resources
- Commitment to scientific knowledge
- Maintaining trust by managing conflicts of interest
- Commitment to professional responsibilities

Medical Professionalism Project 1999

reason. The purpose of morality is to encourage good and discourage bad actions. Implicit in the notion of moral good is that it ought to be positively sought and acted upon, while moral evil is to be avoided.

No account of medical ethics would be complete without consideration of the Hippocratic *Oath*, which has formed the ethical basis of medical practice for well over two thousand years. The Hippocratic tradition did not arise from any specific religious perspective, although it was subsequently adopted by the Jewish, Christian and Islamic Faiths.

The Hippocratic tradition

The best known code of medical ethics is the time-honoured Hippocratic *Oath* (Table 1.4).

The Hippocratic tradition served to differentiate the practice of medicine from quackery and witchcraft. The Greek physician was distinguished from the 'medicine man'. According to the anthropologist Margaret Mead:

'Throughout the primitive world the doctor and the sorcerer tended to be the same person. . . . He who had the power to cure would necessarily be able to kill. Depending on who was paying the bill, the doctor/witch doctor could try to relieve pain or send the patient to another world. Then came a profound change in the consciousness of the medical profession—made both literal and symbolic in the Hippocratic *Oath* . . . For the first time in our tradition there was a complete separation between killing and curing. . . . With the Greeks the distinction was made clear. One profession . . . was to be dedicated completely to life under all circumstances, regardless of rank, age or intellect.'

'The Physician', *Journal of Ethnography* 3, No. 1, 1937.

The doctor–patient relationship from a Hippocratic perspective

In the Hippocratic tradition, the doctor–patient relationship is based on trust. Patients are amongst

Table 1.4 The Hippocratic *Oath*

'According to my ability and judgement I will in every particular keep this oath and covenant. To regard him who teaches this art equally with my parents. To share my substance with him, and, if need be, to relieve his necessities and to regard his offspring equally with my brethren and to teach them this art, if they should wish to learn it, without fee or stipulation. To impart knowledge by precept and by lecture and by every other mode of instruction to my sons, to the sons of my teacher and to pupils who are bound by stipulation and by oath according to the law of medicine but to no other. I will use that regimen which according to my ability and judgement shall be for the welfare of the sick and I will refrain from that which may be baneful or injurious. If any should ask of me a drug to produce death, I will not give it. Nor will I suggest or counsel such. In like manner I will not give a woman a pessary to procure an abortion. With purity and holiness will I watch closely my life and my art. I will not cut for stone but give way to those who are practitioners in this work. Into whatever house I shall enter there I shall go for the benefit of the sick, abstaining from every voluntary act of injustice and corruption and from any act of seduction of man or woman, slave or free.

Whatever in the life of men I shall see or hear in my practice, or without my practice, which should not be made public, I will hold silence thereon, believing such things should not be spoken. While I keep this oath inviolate and unbroken may it be granted me to enjoy my life and my art, forever honoured by men. But should I by transgression violate it, let the reverse be my lot.'

Hippocrates 460–377 BC

the most vulnerable members of society. Illness necessarily places the patient in a situation that requires the doctor to make a diagnosis and provide the appropriate treatment. The relationship is regarded as one of partnership rather than 'paternalism'.

The purpose of medicine — to benefit the sick

In the Hippocratic tradition it is axiomatic that the purpose of medicine is to benefit the sick. While the merits of a particular treatment for a given

patient are a matter of professional judgement, the intrinsic worth of the patient is unquestioned. Hence, while doctors may make a clinical judgement on the benefits of treatment, they are neither qualified nor entitled to make value judgements regarding the moral worth of the individual. Recognition of the intrinsic value of the individual requires respect for all human life and the prohibition of deliberate killing.

Refrain from harm

It is the patient who is being treated, not simply the disease.

'First we must consider the nature of man in general and of each individual and the characteristics of each disease.'

(Hipporates: *Epidemics*)

The doctor must weigh the risks and benefits of treatment and advise what therapy is indicated, avoiding that which would be inappropriate or unduly burdensome.

'Practise two things in your dealings with disease: either help or do not harm the patient.'

(Hippocrates: *Epidemics*)

Indeed, some patients are better off without treatment.

'It is better not to treat those who have internal cancers since, if treated, they die quickly; but if not treated they last a long time.'

(Hippocrates: *Aphorisms*)

Trust and integrity

The trust between doctor and patient requires confidentiality and the integrity of the physician. There is a prohibition against 'any form of wrongdoing, or of any act of seduction of male or female, bond or free'. This aspect of the *Oath* was all the more remarkable in ancient Greek society in view of its general attitude towards women and acceptance of slavery. There is ample evidence of the selflessness and dedication of Greek physicians in the *Epidemics*, where the case histories referred to patients from all walks of life, including rich and poor, citizens and slaves, and visitors from abroad. The same is also seen in Thucydides' account of the plague in Athens, where there was a high mortality amongst doctors treating plague victims.

Fees

In *Precepts*, Hippocrates exhorted physicians to consider the patient's means in fixing fees; they should be prepared to treat some patients for nothing. The advice in his *Decorum* was that 'it is better to reproach patients you have saved than to extort money from those in danger of dying'.

The Hippocratic Oath as a model code of medical ethics

The Hippocratic *Oath* is a duty-based code. It predates Christianity and Islam, but is compatible with both, and also with Judaism. What is particularly conspicuous by its absence is any reference to personal patient autonomy and informed consent. Why the *Oath* should ignore what is now such a modern preoccupation in medical ethics is unclear. One might speculate that the decision to be treated was implied by seeking help in the first place. The Greek physician would certainly have held that he was the 'expert' and that the patient, as a layman, could not have known the nature and prognosis of his illness nor its treatment. Furthermore, treatment would have been limited, except in the fields of basic orthopaedics, trauma, obstetrics and pain relief.

The Hippocratic *Oath* and tradition has formed the basis of medical practice for well over two thousand years. Like the Magna Carta and the Ten Commandments, it is refreshingly short and succinct. It is very doubtful if any contemporary code of medical practice could compete with it,

Medical ethics and religion

Whilst contemporary medical ethics is often seen from a largely secular perspective, the role of the great world religions must not be overlooked. For many doctors, nurses and patients, ethical decision-making has a religious significance, and ethics is indistinguishable from morality. In a multicultural society, clinicians must be aware of the religious sensitivities of their patients and how their beliefs may affect their approach to illness and treatment decisions. A patient's decision to accept or refuse treatment will include considerations beyond the merely clinical. For example, a mother might decide to forgo chemotherapy for cancer during pregnancy in order to protect the foetus.

A brief account is therefore given of how religious belief may affect decision-making by patients. Belief in God and active Church membership statistics are shown in Tables 1.5 and 1.6.
● Atheism is uncommon (10%) and belief in God is found in the majority of Britons (58%).
● The main denomination among active church-goers is Roman Catholic.
● The numbers of adherents of Islam, Hinduism, and Sikhism are on the increase.
A brief outline of the ethical positions and biographies of some of the moral philosophers who have had an important influence on Medical Ethics is outlined in Appendix 1, which also contains some suggestions for further reading for those with a particular interest in theoretical ethics. This appendix is not comprehensive. Nevertheless, it may serve to illustrate the rich heritage of ethical thought behind modern medical ethics, which is a subject that is still in a continuous state of development.

Table 1.5 Belief in God in Great Britain 1998

I know God really exists and I have no doubt about it.	21%
While I have doubts, I feel I do believe in God.	23%
I find myself believing in God at some times, but not at others.	14%
I don't believe in a personal God, but I do believe in a Higher Power of some kind.	14%
I don't know whether there is a God and I don't believe there is any way to find out.	15%
I don't believe in God.	10%
Not answered	3%

Source: National Centre for Social Research: *British Social Attitudes Survey*.

Table 1.6 Active Church Membership (thousands)

	1980	1990	1995
Trinitarian Churches			
Roman Catholic	2,457	2,201	1,915
Anglican	2,179	1,728	1,785
Presbyterian	1,438	1,214	1,100
Other free Churches	516	601	648
Methodist	521	452	401
Orthodox	203	266	289
Baptist	240	231	223
Non-Trinitarian Churches			
Mormons	114	160	171
Jehovah's Witnesses	85	117	131
Other non-Trinitarian	154	182	220
Other Religions			
Muslim	306	495	580
Sikh	150	250	350
Hindu	120	140	155
Jewish	111	101	94
Others	53	87	116

Source: 'Church Membership' in *Social Trends* 29. 1999 (www.dti.gov.uk)

Table 1.7 Summary of Protestant bioethics

Mainstream Protestant ethics accepts:
- the sovereignty of God;
- the value of free will and personal autonomy;
- the concept of medicine as a vocation as well as a profession;
- the importance of Scripture (the Bible) as a source of ethics.

However, views may well differ on:
- abortion, contraception, genetic testing, and reproductive technology; and
- end-of-life issues.

Certain denominations do have specific beliefs and practices in relation to medical care; hence:
- Jehovah's Witnesses may refuse blood transfusions; and
- Christian Scientists may decline conventional medical treatment.

Traditional ethical theories

There are three main ethical theories that have preoccupied moral philosophers. All three theories have been adapted to the study of ethical behaviour within a healthcare context that has become known as 'bioethics'. They are not necessarily mutually exclusive:

- Deontological theories
- Utilitarianism
- Virtue ethics.

Deontological theories

Deontological ethics are duty-based (from the Greek *deon*, meaning 'it is necessary'), with an emphasis on the fulfilment of obligations. Deontology seeks a general basis for our duties and obligations that rest upon fundamental principles. Religiously-based systems are deontological, and rest on belief in God. However, the German philosopher Kant advocated a deontological system that did not require religious belief, though it did not exclude it. His famous 'categorical impera-

tive' states that one ought to 'act only on that maxim that can at the same time become a universal law'. This is an expression of the 'principle of universalizability', which requires that whatever principles of action one proposes ought to be generally applicable ('universalizable'). The categorical imperative is not so much a source as a test of moral principles. Appeals to universal principles obviate claims of arbitrariness in decision-making. An example of a universalizable imperative is 'do unto others as you would have them do unto you', which mirrors the Christian command 'Love thy neighbour as thyself.' Another moral injunction expressed as a categorical imperative is 'Thou shall not kill' (*Exodus* 20:13).

Christian bioethics

Protestant bioethics (Table 1.7)

Protestantism applies to a number of non-Catholic Christian denominations with a wide range of ethical beliefs. Hence, it is not possible to define a uniquely Protestant medical ethic.

Historically Protestantism has stressed respect for persons, the freedom of the individual and personal autonomy. Most Protestants would argue that autonomy can only be fully expressed within the context of a relationship with God. The doctor–patient relationship can also be viewed in relation to the concepts of vocation and ministry to others. The work of the Salvation Army is a clear example of such ministry.

The range of ethical stands taken by Protestant ethicists has been very broad. Paul Ramsey advocated a deontological approach involving unexceptional moral principles. His views on the value of the individual and the 'canon of loyalty' that should exist between doctor and patients have been very influential. Joseph Fletcher proposed a situation ethics resembling act-utilitarianism. He stressed the need to view ethical issues from the patient's perspective and the importance of freedom and choice. James Gustafson described how ethical reflections should begin in the light of ordinary human existence. Religious beliefs and assumptions might then influence the evaluation of a given clinical situation and the weight that should be given to particular values and the consequences of actions. Doctors will need to be particularly sensitive in dealing with the wide spectrum of views and beliefs that may be encountered amongst their Protestant patients.

Protestant attitudes to death and dying

A special ministry may be expected, depending on the particular tradition. It is wise to consult relatives and friends. Baptism or Prayers of Blessing for infants in danger of dying may be offered. There are usually no objections to organ donation or post-mortems. Both burial and cremation are generally acceptable.

Roman Catholic bioethics (Table 1.8)

The Roman Catholic Church constitutes the largest Christian denomination worldwide. It remains one of the most important providers of healthcare across the world. The Catholic tradition is derived from:
- Scripture.
- The authoritative interpretation of Scripture by the official teaching office of the Church, consisting of all the bishops in communion with the chief

Table 1.8 Summary of Roman Catholic bioethics

Central to Catholic bioethics is:
- belief in the sanctity of life from conception to natural death; and
- the concept of the person as a composite of body and soul.

This implies a duty to preserve life by all 'ordinary' means.

There is therefore a prohibition of:
- Direct abortion
- Artificial contraception
- Abortifacient drugs and devices
- IVF
- Destructive experiments on the foetus
- Suicide
- Euthanasia by deliberate act or omission

bishop (called the Pope) in a consistent line stretching back to the first chief bishop, St Peter.
- The writings of the approved theologians and teachers (called 'Doctors of the Church'), such as St. Thomas Aquinas.
- Catholic ethics is concerned with a range of issues, including the right to health care, the duty to preserve life and the limits of that duty, human procreation, reproductive technology and end-of-life decisions. The Roman Catholic Church has made explicit statements on all of these issues as part of its official teaching. Catholic medical ethics is compatible with the Hippocratic tradition.

Central to Catholic bioethics is a belief in the sanctity of life and the concept of the person as a composite of body and soul.

In common with the other monotheistic religions of Judaism and Islam, Christianity maintains that there is a duty to protect innocent human life. There is therefore a moral obligation to provide and accept all ordinary means of preserving life. Suicide and euthanasia are forbidden within the Catholic tradition, as in other traditions. Extraordinary means of treatment have been defined as those that are associated with excessive risk, pain, or expenditure, or would not provide a reasonable hope of benefit to the patient. Catholics are not obliged to accept 'extraordinary means' of treatment.

Catholic attitudes to death and dying

Catholic patients will appreciate spiritual support at the end of life, including Holy Communion, the Sacrament of Reconciliation (Confession) and the Last Rites. It is appropriate to consider calling a priest when death is imminent. Infants and babies in danger of death should be baptized.

There is no objection to organ donation, post mortem examinations or cremation.

Eastern and Oriental Orthodox and Catholic Christians

There are a great many other Christian denominations that are neither Roman Catholic nor Protestant, of which the majority are probably the Eastern and Oriental Orthodox and Catholic Churches.

By and large these Churches have very similar bioethical beliefs to those of Roman Catholics, although there are some differences among the Orthodox Churches.

The chief differences are theological and liturgical (i.e. ritual), but doctors must take care not to assume that the beliefs of patients from these traditions are the same as those of Roman Catholics, as this can cause offence and upset to them.

Islamic bioethics (Table 1.9)

Islamic bioethics arises from a framework of values based upon revelation and tradition. It is linked to the teachings of the Qu'ran, and is based upon a combination of principles, duties and rights and a call to virtue (*Ihsan*). It emphasizes preventive

Table 1.9 Summary of Islamic bioethics

Central to Islamic bioethics are:
- A belief that human beings are the crown of God's creation
- A respect for patients—all human life has value
- The Hippocratic tradition
- A duty to respect all patients and treat them with compassion
- A duty to protect life in all its stages and in all circumstances
- The prohibition of direct killing

medicine as a means to continued health. Islam holds that patients must be treated with respect and compassion, taking into account the physical, mental and spiritual dimensions of illness. Because of their common Mosaic heritage, it holds in common many fundamental values with Judaism and Christianity, and shares with them a similar code of morality.

Human beings are seen as the crown of God's creation. They are endowed with reason, choice and responsibilities, including stewardship over their own health, the environment and all other creatures. While illness is seen as a trial or even as a cleansing ordeal, it is not a curse or punishment. Patients are obliged to seek treatment and to avoid fatalism.

The Hippocratic tradition is acknowledged by Islam. The code of ethics of the physician Al-Tabari, written in AD 970, describes the characteristics of the physician and his duties to his patients, to colleagues and to the community. The Hippocratic ideal is clearly seen in this code and also in the 1981 Islamic Code of Medical Ethics (see further reading section on Chapter 1 in Appendix 2). Life has value even if it is of poor quality. The taking of life is regarded as a grave sin. 'Whosoever killeth a human being . . . it shall be as if he had killed all humankind, and whosoever saveth the life of one, it shall be as if he saved the life of all humankind' (Qu'ran 5:32).

The Oath of the Muslim Doctor has an undertaking 'to protect human life in all stages and under all circumstances, doing [one's] utmost to rescue it from death, malady, pain and anxiety. To be, all the way, an instrument of God's mercy, extending . . . medical care to near and far, virtuous and sinner and friend and enemy.'

The Qu'ran has a surprising amount of accurate detail concerning human embryology that underlies the Islamic appreciation of the ethical and moral status of the embryo and the foetus before birth.

Muslim attitudes to death and dying

The patient may wish to sit or lie facing Mecca. Friends may want to be with the patient reading the Qu'ran. After death the body should be wrapped in one or two plain white sheets. The foot of the bed should be facing Mecca or the patient should be turned on their right side so that the face looks towards the Holy City. The body should not be washed in hospital and the nails or hair should not be cut. The central Mosque should be contacted and will handle washing of the body and organize prayers at the Mosque. Muslims may oppose post mortem examinations unless they are required by law. Donations of organs are generally allowed with the permission of those concerned. Cremation is forbidden in Islam.

Jewish medical ethics (Table 1.10)

Jewish bioethics applies the principles of Jewish law (*Halacha*), the Torah (written law) and the Talmud (oral law) to ethical problems. Judaic bioethics is a duty-based system with particular emphasis on good deeds (*mitzvoth*) within the context of relationships. A further important source of Jewish legal authority is the *Responsa* literature, consisting of opinions of scholars over the last 2,000 years. In practice, a Rabbi may serve as an 'expert counsellor' to a physician or patient, interpreting Halachic law in relation to a given problem or ethical dilemma.

Several foundation tenets underlie much of Jewish bioethics:
- Human life has infinite value.
- Ageing, illness and death are a natural part of life.
- Improvement of the patient's quality of life is a constant commitment.
- Human beings are to act as responsible stewards

in preserving their bodies, which belong to God.
- Short of committing murder, incest or public idolatry, they may violate any other law in order to save human life. Hence, the duty to treat illness or preserve health overrides any presumed right to withhold treatment or commit suicide.
- Traditional Judaism prohibits suicide, euthanasia, the withholding or withdrawing of life-preserving treatment, and abortion when the mother's life or health is not at risk. However, one need not impede or hinder the process of dying once it has begun.

Jewish attitudes to death and dying

Dying patients should not be left alone, and relatives may wish to stay. There should be an opportunity for saying a Prayer of Confession and to receive an Affirmation of Faith—which can be said by relatives. The patient's own Rabbi should normally be called first before the contact Rabbi.

After death the nearest relatives may wish to close the eyes. The arms should be extended and the hands open. The body should be touched as little as possible. The body should be left if death occurs during the Sabbath, and the advice of relatives should be sought. The body should be wrapped in a plain white sheet, and the relatives may wish to keep vigil. Burial should usually occur within 24 hours if possible.

Hinduism and Sikhism (Table 1.11)

Both Hinduism and Sikhism take a duty-based,

Table 1.10 Summary of Jewish bioethics

Central beliefs in Jewish bioethics:
- Human life has infinite value and belongs to God.
- Doctors have a duty to act as responsible stewards to preserve life, which belongs to God, whilst accepting that death is inevitable.

Judaism prohibits:
- Suicide, including physician-assisted suicide.
- Euthanasia, including deliberately withholding treatment so as to cause death.
- Abortion when the mother's life is not at risk.

Table 1.11 Summary of bioethics in Hinduism and Sikhism

Central to Hinduism and Sikhism is a belief in rebirth.
 Hinduism and Sikhism:
- have a duty-based approach to bioethics;
- take a holistic view of the person;
- value family, culture, spirituality and the environment.

There is
- a duty to maintain a lifestyle conducive to physical and mental well-being;
- a rejection of abortion, except to save the mother's life;
- an emphasis on purity and cleanliness;
- a holistic approach to consent.

rather than rights-based approach to ethics. Indeed, there is no word for 'rights' in the traditional Hindu and Sikh languages. Both Hindus and Sikhs believe that life, birth and death are repeated for each person. What happens in life has a bearing on future lives. Both good and evil thoughts and actions leave a trace in the unconscious that is carried forward into the next life. *Karma* rejects any absolute beginning of life. The moment of conception is the rebirth of a person who has had many previous lives. Abortion sends the soul back into the karmic cycle of rebirth, and is regarded as murder at any stage of foetal development, although it may be accepted in order to save the life of the mother.

Hinduism and Sikhism take a holistic view of the person that values the importance of family, culture, the environment and spirituality. Traditional teachings deal with the duties of individuals and families to maintain a lifestyle conducive to physical and mental well-being. The individual is not seen as autonomous but rather as integrated into family, caste and environment. Hence consent has to be seen in holistic terms within a particular cultural context that includes a spiritual dimension. Decision-making may therefore have to be negotiated with the family spokesman. There is a strong male predominance in questions of consent.

The emphasis on purity and cleanliness must be respected, and may mean that women will prefer to be seen and examined by women doctors. An older Hindu or Sikh woman may be the best interpreter for urological and gynaecological matters, especially if she understands medical terminology. Whilst in hospital the Hindu family may wish to be with the patient all the time.

Hindu attitudes to death and dying: *puja* or last rites

Hindu patients may wish to die at home. Death in hospital may be distressing for the relatives. Before death there will be a desire for gifts of food and articles for use by the needy, religious persons and the Temple. Such gifts will be brought by the relatives for the patient to touch. Hindu patients may like to have the leaves of the sacred Tulsi plant and Ganges water placed in their mouth before death. Therefore it is important to notify the relatives if death is imminent.

The family should be consulted as to whether they wish to perform the Last Rites in hospital. These include washing the patient in water mixed with water from the Ganges. Sacred threads or jewellery should not be removed, and the family should be consulted before touching the body. Hindus have no objection to transplantation, but post mortems are not generally welcomed. However, if these latter are required by law, the organs should be returned before the funeral, which should normally occur within 24 hours of death. Hindus are cremated, not buried.

Sikh attitudes to death and dying

A separate room for the dying will be appreciated. The family may wish to say or sing prayers, or taped hymns or prayers may be placed by the patient. Sikh men should always wear five Kakars (the 5 Ks). After death do not remove the five Ks, which are personal objects sacred to Sikhs: the *Kesh*, or unshorn hair—do not cut the hair or beard or remove the turban; the *Kanga* or comb, which is used to fix the uncut hair; the *Kara* or steel bracelet; the *Kachha* or special shorts; and the *Kirpan* or miniature sword. After death the religious symbol, the *Khanda*, is placed on the altar, which in turn should be placed close to the deceased's head. Sikhs are always cremated.

Utilitarianism

For the utilitarian, the morality of actions is to be judged by their utility or usefulness to the majority of people.

The best known form of Utilitarianism is that of Jeremy Bentham, which was developed further by John Stuart Mill, Henry Sidgwick and, latterly, Peter Singer. Bentham argued that actions should aim at producing the greatest good for the greatest number by maximizing pleasure and minimizing pain.

There are several forms of utilitarianism:
• *Classic utilitarianism* judges the consequences of particular acts—'act utilitarianism'.

- *Rule utilitarianism* refers to the overall consequences of following particular rules of conduct. Hence telling lies is considered generally bad because it leads to dishonesty, ignorance or lack of trust. However, in particular cases it might seem to be of benefit, for example, when a lie is told to protect someone from harm.
- *Preference utilitarianism* seeks to maximize an individual's preferences or choices, e.g. something is right for someone because that is what they would want.

The problem of altruism

One problem for utilitarianism in clinical practice is how to explain altruism. Medicine is essentially altruistic, and utilitarian medical ethics must give a reason for helping others. Altruism sometimes seems difficult to justify on the basis of utilitarianism, except that, on balance, if people are generally helpful to others rather than selfish, all tend to benefit. Hence, the maxim 'do unto others as you would have them do unto you' has indirect benefit even if it means sacrificing oneself for others now in the hope of personal gain in the future. John Stuart Mill argued that the standard of utilitarianism 'is not the agent's own greatest happiness, but the greatest amount of happiness altogether, and if it may possibly be doubted whether a noble character is always happier for its nobleness, there can be no doubt that it makes other people happier, and that the world in general is immensely a gainer by it.'

Virtue ethics

Virtue ethics emphasizes the development of character traits that will enable us to become the sort of person who will make right decisions. As such it is consistent with religious ethics.

The ancient Greek philosopher Aristotle divided these traits, or virtues, into moral and intellectual virtues.

Moral virtues included:
- Courage
- Friendship
- Temperance

- Patience
- Truthfulness.

Intellectual virtues included:
- Wisdom
- Right judgement
- Prudence.

Decision-making applied the Golden Mean, or a balance between opposite extremes. For example the moral virtue of courage lies between recklessness on the one hand and foolhardiness on the other.

Virtue ethics was later developed by St Thomas Aquinas in a Christian context. Aquinas also stressed the type of character that we become through our moral actions—e.g. thieves become more dishonest and murderers more callous through their crimes.

Virtue ethics stresses the effects of any moral action, not only on those affected, but also on the moral agents themselves. Hence a kindly, sympathetic doctor will benefit his patients, who experience his empathy, and also become a better person himself by acting generously towards his patients. Such a doctor is also more likely to gain their trust and obtain a better medical history than a callous doctor who, by being curt and abrupt with patients, will become more insensitive and impatient with time. Callousness begets insensitivity and impatience.

Ethical methodology

In recent years there have been attempts to look at the way that ethical decisions are made, i.e. ethical methodology, as a means of 'working through' ethical problems. Most of these have attempted to be less 'value-dependent' than the traditional approaches outlined above. Whether 'value-free' ethics is really possible, or indeed philosophically and logically coherent, is deeply controversial. There are essentially four approaches to such methodology.
- The 'four principles' approach, or Principlism
- Casuistry (case-based reasoning)
- Communitarian Bioethics
- 'Post-modern' Ethics

The 'four principles' approach: Principlism (Beauchamp and Childress)

Advanced by Beauchamp and Childress, this system attempts to balance four principles in deciding any moral issue. The four principles are:

- Respect for patient autonomy
- Beneficence
- Non-maleficence
- Justice.

In some instances, the application of these four principles is easy; in others it is more problematic, and clearly cannot be 'value-free'. Beauchamp and Childress do not allow any appeal to any overarching moral framework for such a balancing judgement. Theirs is a 'principle-based, common morality theory', in which 'some intuitive and subjective weighting are unavoidable, just as they are everywhere in life when we must balance competing goods'. Nevertheless, they argue that such a balancing exercise 'is a process of justification only if adequate reasons are presented'.

One example of Principlism is that of the HIV patient who does not wish to be told the results of an HIV test that comes back positive. Patient autonomy means respecting the patient's wish to remain in ignorance of his HIV status, even though this would place his sexual partners at risk of a potentially fatal sexually transmitted disease. Beauchamp and Childress answer this particular dilemma in one sentence: 'In light of the possible consequences, the disclosure was justified despite the fact that the patient did not want the information.'

Casuistry (case-based reasoning)

Casuistry refers to case-based reasoning. It usually involves the application of general principles to particular cases. However, for others casuistry means that 'the circumstances make the case'. Ethical reasoning then proceeds by the use of analogy, using clear-cut or paradigm examples to decide more complex cases.

For example, how far is it necessary to pursue ineffective curative treatment ('relentless therapy')

in the case of the terminally ill in preference to palliative care?

According to Judaeo-Christian and Islamic ethics it might be argued that:

- It is wrong to kill the patient intentionally, as this would offend the Sanctity of Life Principle.
- It is right to relieve suffering through palliative care.
- 'Extraordinary' means of preserving life are not mandatory (Catholicism).
- It is wrong to interfere with the dying process (Judaism).

From a utilitarian perspective relentless therapy:

- should be judged by its consequences for the patient;
- would add to the patient's misery rather than happiness by increasing suffering;
- is medically futile; and hence
- should be replaced by good palliative care to reduce suffering.

Taking a 'principlist' approach:

- Relentless therapy would maximize maleficence by increasing patient suffering.
- Palliative care would maximize beneficence by relieving distressing symptoms.
- Respect for patient autonomy means involving the patient as much as possible in their treatment.
- Palliative care does not involve intentional killing, and hence does not offend justice.

Hence, taking all three approaches, relentless therapy would be stopped in favour of palliative care. However, the ethical reasoning is different.

Communitarian bioethics

Communitarian ethics assumes that ethics is linked to wider political and social considerations. In a pluralistic society there may be few shared values and also few conceptual frameworks and resources to meet ethical demands. Communitarians believe that it is necessary to restore shared values, otherwise members of society will always be talking at cross purposes. Clarity will only be achieved through dialogue. Alasdair MacIntyre, for example, pointed to the divergence of opinion surrounding 'hard cases' such as abortion.

'Post-modern' ethics

The most important aspect of 'post-modern ethics' is the belief that there are no moral absolutes. It has been termed a 'celebration of moral relativism'.

For the 'post-modernist' there has been a loss of traditional ethical values coupled with an increasing plurality of ethical views within society. There are no 'moral signposts'. We will need to rely upon greater self-monitoring and self-evaluation. This may even have encouraged the move to greater external regulation of medical practice. As medical ethics decline, medical law increases. Hence, it has been suggested that across a wide range of medical practice, such as human research, the rationing of healthcare, organ procurement and transplantation, reproductive technology, and questions of withdrawing and withholding life-preserving treatment, decisions are reached through explicit rules, protocols and guidelines. From a 'post-modern' standpoint ethical conclusions are 'constructed' rather than derived through philosophical reflection. Complex issues may be 'decided' by relatively few individuals. This is clearly seen in the field of reproductive technology, where a small number of unelected individuals in the Human Fertilization and Embryology Authority make decisions that profoundly affect human embryonic research and fertility treatment.

Keypoints

- Ethical considerations are essential to the practice of medicine.
- The principles underlying the Hippocratic tradition remain central to bioethics.
- It is important to recognize the moral and cultural sensitivities of patients, especially in relation to death and dying.

Chapter 2

Sources of medical law

Civil and criminal law

Medical law includes both the civil and, less commonly, the criminal law.

Civil law

- The function of civil law is to redress the infringement of legal rights.
- Successful civil litigation may lead to an injunction preventing, or requiring, a certain action or may lead to the award of monetary compensation known as 'damages'.
- The standard of proof in a civil case is 'on the balance of probabilities' whereas in criminal law it is 'beyond reasonable doubt' (The General Medical Council adopts the criminal standard of proof in cases of serious professional misconduct.)

Criminal law

- Crime involves the infringement of laws that have been enacted by the State to govern the way people should behave.
- Criminal matters are investigated by the police and referred to the Crown Prosecution Service. The legal remedy for criminal activity is punishment in the form of fines or imprisonment.
- For a crime to be committed there must be both the *actus reus*, or guilty act, and the *mens rea*, or guilty mind. Hence, the *actus reus* is the act or omission that constitutes the crime itself and the *mens rea* is the mental element or intention behind the crime. This is embodied in the dictum *Actus non facit reum nisi mens sit rea* ('There cannot be a guilty act unless there is a guilty mind.')

Healthcare workers are rarely accused of criminal activity in their work. However some actions might give rise to either a criminal or civil action, for example the case of *R v Adokamo* (Table 2.2).

Developments in the law: the roles of statute and common law

Legal developments occur either through changes in statute law or by means of statutory instruments enacted through Parliament, or through decisions made in the courts by judges.

Table 2.1 Civil Law and Criminal Law cases

Civil law cases	Criminal law cases
Cases are begun by a 'Claim'.	Cases are 'prosecuted'.
Cases involve disputes between individuals or organizations.	Cases involve breaking the rules governing society (a crime is a 'public' wrong).
Cases are brought by claimants against a defendant.	Cases are brought by a prosecutor—usually the Prosecution Service—on behalf of the Crown.
Defendants remain free before trial.	Defendants may be held in custody or may be out on bail.
Cases are usually tried without a jury.	Trial by jury for more serious crimes. Minor offences are tried by magistrates.
Does not usually require demonstration of 'guilt'.	Requires *mens rea* and *actus reus* (guilty mind and guilty act).
Cases decided on 'balance of probability.	Cases decided on proof 'beyond reasonable doubt'.
Remedy is usually compensation through damages or injunction to prevent further harm.	Punished by fines, community service or imprisonment.
Examples: law of contract; property law; family law; tort law (a tort is a civil wrong, e.g. trespass, negligence, libel).	Examples: murder, manslaughter, theft, assault and battery.

Table 2.2 Manslaughter through gross negligence

An anaesthetist failed to notice that the oxygen supply to the patient had been discontinued for around six minutes during an eye operation. The patient suffered a fatal cardiac arrest. The anaesthetist was found to have been so grossly negligent as to be guilty of manslaughter. The defendant appealed and his conviction was upheld by the House of Lords. According to Lord McKay 'You should only convict a doctor of causing death by negligence if you think he did something which no reasonably skilled doctor should have done.'

R v. Adomako (1994)

Statute law is passed by Parliament according to the democratic process.

• Acts of Parliament constitute primary legislation.

• Regulations and Orders are usually brought into being by Statutory Instruments, which can be brought into law by Ministers of the Crown under powers given to them by primary legislation.

• Statutory Instruments, Regulations and Orders are sometimes called 'delegated legislation' or 'secondary legislation'.

Common Law is developed through decisions made by judges according to precedent, so that legal principles established in one case must be applied in similar future cases in lower courts. There is a hierarchy of authority within the judicial system, with the House of Lords taking precedence over the Court of Appeal, the High Court, the County Court and the Magistrates' courts.

Certain aspects of medical law are governed largely by statute law. As we shall discover in a later chapter, abortion is governed mainly by the Abortion Act 1967. Conversely, the law in relation to clinical negligence has developed chiefly through case law. The standard of negligence established in the *Bolam* test (*Bolam v Friern HMC (1957)*) was derived through common law, not statute.

Since October 2000, the Human Rights (1998) Act has incorporated the European Convention on Human Rights into UK domestic law. However, interpretation of the European Convention on Human Rights may differ between countries. For example, the interpretation made by a domestic court in France would not be binding in England, and might even deviate from principles decided in England. The English system of binding precedent is not applied in the same way in Europe, and thus only the decisions of English and Welsh courts bind in England and Wales. Other courts' verdicts are merely persuasive.

Increasingly, the courts are being used to provide 'declaratory relief' concerning the lawfulness or otherwise of particular medical procedures such as the withdrawal of hydration and nutrition, non-therapeutic sterilization, the performance of a Caesarean section or the administration of blood transfusions. That simply means that the court 'declares' what the law is in each case, so that doctors and hospital administrations can act with immunity and safety by following the decision of the court.

The Human Rights Act 1998

Background

The United Kingdom was one of the first signatories to the European Convention on Human Rights and Fundamental Freedoms (the Convention) in 1951. However, it was not until 1998 that the Human Rights Act was passed by Parliament so that the Convention was incorporated into domestic law. This means that all courts are required to decide cases in a way that is compatible with Convention rights unless they are prevented from so doing by primary legislation. The Act contains new rights that are directly enforceable against public bodies, such as Health Authorities and Hospital Trusts. The Act cannot be used to override primary legislation, but courts have the power to issue 'declarations of incompatibility', and there is a fast-track procedure for governments to remedy such incompatibility.

Convention Rights

Article 2: the right to life

Article 2 reads:
● Everyone's right to life shall be protected by law. No one shall be deprived of his life intentionally save in the execution of a sentence of a court following his conviction of a crime for which this penalty is provided by law.
● Deprivation of life shall not be regarded as inflicted in contravention of this article when it results from the use of force which is no more than absolutely necessary:
  ● in defence of any person from unlawful violence;
  ● in order to effect a lawful arrest or to prevent the escape of a person lawfully detained;
  ● in action lawfully taken for the purpose of quelling a riot or insurrection.

Article 2 has been described as 'one of the most fundamental provisions of the Convention'. The Commission has established that Article 2 not only means that the state must 'not only refrain from taking life "intentionally" but, further, take appropriate steps to safeguard life'.

The second paragraph of Article 2 details the exceptions to the right to life. All the exceptions are involved with the maintaining of law and order and self-defence. However, while Article 2 does not prohibit the execution of a death sentence, Protocol 6 now requires the abolition of the death penalty.

The Court at Strasbourg held that Article 2 is not limited to situations of gross negligence or wilful disregard of life. In the case of *Osman v United Kingdom* (1999), the police failed to protect Ahmed Osman from being killed by a known paedophile. An action for negligence against the police was dismissed. It was held that it would be unreasonable and unfair to hold that the police could be liable for failing to protect potential victims from unpredictable crimes. The court said:

'The Court does not accept the government's view that the failure to perceive the risk to life in the circumstances known at the time or to take preventative measures to avoid that risk must be tantamount to gross negligence or wilful disregard of the duty to protect life . . . it is sufficient for an applicant to show that the authorities did not do all that could be reasonably expected of them to avoid a real and immediate risk to life of which they have or ought to have knowledge.'

Article 2 may therefore be relevant in relation to such matters as:
● Abortion, including partial birth abortion
● Life-saving operations and treatment
● 'Do not resuscitate' orders
● Withholding hydration and nutrition from PVS patients
● Access to treatment and 'postcode' prescribing
● Ensuring competence of medical practitioners and avoiding medical negligence.

In the case of *Ireland v United Kingdom* (1978) the court in Strasbourg examined five techniques used by the British in Northern Ireland to interrogate prisoners who had allegedly been involved in acts of terrorism. The activities prohibited by Article 3 were defined as:

- Torture: deliberate inhumane treatment causing very serious and cruel suffering.
- Inhuman treatment: treatment that causes intense physical and mental suffering.
- Degrading treatment: treatment that arouses in the victim a feeling of fear, anguish and inferiority capable of humiliating and debasing the victim and possibly breaking his or her physical or moral resistance.

Article 3: freedom from torture and inhuman or degrading treatment

Article 3 reads:
No one shall be subjected to torture or to inhuman or degrading treatment or punishment.

Article 5: right to liberty and security of person

Article 5 reads:
- Everyone has the right to liberty and security of person. No one shall be deprived of his liberty save in the following cases and in accordance with a procedure prescribed by law . . . [*the cases are thereafter set out*]
- Everyone who is arrested shall be informed promptly, in a language which he understands, of the reasons for his arrest and of any charge against him.
- Everyone arrested or detained in accordance with the provisions of paragraph 1(c) of this article shall be brought promptly before a judge or other officer authorized by law to exercise a judicial power and shall be entitled to trial within a reasonable time or to release pending a trial. Release may be conditioned by guarantees to appear for trial.
- Everyone who is deprived of his liberty by arrest or detention shall be entitled to take proceedings by which the lawfulness of his detention shall be decided speedily by a court and his release ordered if the detention is not lawful.
- Everyone who has been the victim of arrest or detention in contravention of the provisions of this article shall have an enforceable right to compensation.

Cases involving infringements of Article 3 have included rape committed by soldiers, racial discrimination, deportation with risks of ill-treatment in the receiving country or deportation with the risk of inadequate medical treatment for AIDS in the receiving country. Physical abuse by police has also been an issue under Article 3, as has 'the infliction of mental suffering by creating a state of anguish and stress by means other than bodily assault'.

Article 3 might be invoked in future to deal with such medical matters as:
- Delays in diagnosis or treatment
- 'Trolley waits' in A&E wards
- Inadequate palliative care
- Poor standards of care within hospitals and institutions and by Social Services
- Experimental and non-consensual treatment
- The rationing of healthcare and 'postcode prescribing'.

The deprivation of an individual's freedom is always a serious matter. Article 5 will be of major importance to psychiatrists in relation to the compulsory admission of patients for assessment and treatment under the Mental Health Act. It will also need to be taken into consideration in relation to the proposed reform of mental health legislation.

Under Article 5, the 'right to liberty' and 'security of the person' is protected by four principles:
- No one shall be deprived of their liberty except in accordance with a procedure prescribed by law.
- The only grounds for deprivation of liberty are specifically set out in 5(1)(a) to (f). This list is meant to be exhaustive.
- Anyone subject to detention can challenge the legality of their detention.
- Detention in contravention of Article 5 entitles the person to compensation.

Article 5(1)(e) allows the detention of those with infectious diseases, persons of unsound mind, alcoholics, drug addicts and vagrants. Such people may be 'considered as occasionally dangerous for public safety', or 'their own interests may necessitate their detention'.

Under Article 6, various issues could be raised:
• Independence of the Health and Conduct Committees of the GMC
• Delays before the hearing of negligence claims against doctors
• Delays in access to review by Mental Health tribunals

Article 6: right to a fair trial

Article 6 reads:
• In the determination of his civil rights and obligations or of any criminal charge against him, everyone is entitled to a fair and public hearing within a reasonable time by an independent and impartial tribunal established by law. Judgment shall be pronounced publicly but the press and public may be excluded from all or part of the trial in the interests of morals, public order or national security in a democratic society, where the interests of juveniles or the protection of the private life of the parties so require, or to the extent strictly necessary in the opinion of the court in special circumstances where publicity would prejudice the interests of justice.
• Everyone charged with a criminal offence shall be presumed innocent until proved guilty according to law.
• Everyone charged with a criminal offence has the following minimal rights:
   • to be informed promptly, in a language which he understands and in detail, of the nature and cause of the accusation against him;
   • to have adequate time and facilities for the preparation of his defence;
   • to defend himself in person or through legal assistance of his own choosing or, if he has not sufficient means to pay for legal assistance, to be given it free when the interests of justice so require;
   • to examine or have examined witnesses against him and to obtain the attendance and examination of witnesses on his behalf under the same conditions as witnesses against him; and
   • to have the free assistance of an interpreter if he cannot understand or speak the language used in court.

• The right to legal aid (now simply called 'Public Funding')

• The right to a public hearing in medical disciplinary hearings
• The need to undergo trial within a reasonable period of the alleged offence.

Article 8: right to respect for private and family life

Article 8 reads:
Everyone has the right to respect for his private and family life, his home and his correspondence . . .

The bulk of the case law here is concerned with the definitions of 'private life', 'home' and 'correspondence'.

Under Article 8, issues that may be of medical significance include:
• Sexual activities as an element of private life
• Age of consent
• Sadomasochistic activity

Article 9: freedom of thought, conscience and religion

Article 9 reads:
Everyone has the right to freedom of thought, conscience and religion; this right includes freedom to change his religion or belief and freedom, either alone or in community with others and in public and private, to manifest his religion or belief, in worship, teaching, practice and observance . . .

This Article might be invoked in relation to conscientious objection to abortion on social grounds, circumcision, and the administration of blood and blood products to Jehovah's Witnesses. Religious beliefs might also need to be taken into consideration if ever the use of tissue from cloned human embryos becomes a practical reality.
• The recognition of homosexual and transsexual unions
• The Data Protection Act 1998
• Confidentiality of medical records
• Divorce
• Care proceedings
• Adoption
• Contact with children.

Article 10: freedom of expression
Article 10 reads:
Everyone has the right to freedom of expression. This right shall include freedom to hold opinions and to receive and impart information and ideas without interference by public authority and regardless of frontiers. This Article shall not prevent States from requiring the licensing of broadcasting, television or cinema enterprises . . .

Article 10 might be applicable to:
- 'Whistle blowing'
- Doctors' advertising
- Advising or counselling women in relation to abortion.

Table 2.3 Significance of Articles of Human Rights Act 1988 to medical practice

Article	Issue	Clinical implications
2	'Right to life'	Suicide, euthanasia, abortion, partial birth abortion, 'Do not resuscitate' orders.
		Withholding and withdrawing life-sustaining treatment.
		Access to healthcare; postcode prescribing.
3	'Inhumane and degrading treatment'	Delays in treatment and diagnosis.
		Inadequate care, e.g. inadequate palliation.
		Experimental and non-consensual treatment, e.g. in psychiatric therapy.
		Forced feeding.
		Rationing of healthcare.
5	'Liberty and security of the person'	Psychiatric detentions.
		Compulsory treatment under mental health law.
6	'Right to a fair trial'	GMC and disciplinary proceedings.
		Complaints procedures.
		Clinical negligence cases.
		Hearings not held within a reasonable period.
		The right to be made aware of the nature of allegations against one.
		Standards of proof of allegations required.
		Access to Mental Health Tribunals.
8	'Respect for private and family life'	Sexual activities (private life).
		Data Protection (confidentiality).
		Divorce, care proceedings, adoption.
		Knowledge of genetic parents.
		Reproductive issues (IVF, AID).
9	'Freedom of thought, conscience and religion'	Conscientious objection to abortion and euthanasia.
10	'Freedom of expression'	Advertising.
		'Whistle-blowing'.
		Right to comment on health issues.
12	'Right to marry and found a family'	Same-sex 'marriages'.
		Access to reproductive technology.
		Laws in relation to the regulation of reproductive technology, e.g. the extent of the jurisdiction of the HFEA.
14	'Prohibition of discrimination'	Employment issues.
		Trade union membership.
		Discrimination in relation to gender, age or disability.
		Bullying and harassment of staff.

Article 12: right to marry and found a family

Article 12 reads:

Men and women of marriageable age have the right to marry and to found a family, according to the national laws governing the exercise of this right.

The scope of Article 12 is much narrower than that of Article 8 and is concerned with procreation within the traditional family unit.

'The right to marry guaranteed by Article 12 refers to the traditional marriage between persons of the opposite sex. This appears from the wording of the article, which makes it clear that Article 12 is mainly concerned to protect marriage as the basis of the family.'

Rees v United Kingdom (1986)

Article 12 is restricted 'according to national laws'. Hence, Diane Blood was allowed to use her dead husband's sperm to conceive a child on the basis of the European Union's free movement law rather than that of Article 12 of the Convention.

Article 14: prohibition of discrimination

Article 14 reads:

The enjoyment of the rights and freedoms set forth in this Convention shall be secured without discrimination on any ground such as sex, race, colour, language, religion, political or other opinion, national or social origin, association with a national minority, property, birth or other status.

Article 14 is not an 'equal treatment guarantee'. It does however require equal access to Convention rights.

Grounds for discrimination identified by the Court and Commission have included matters relating to:

- Sex, marital status, sexual orientation, and birth outside marriage;
- Membership of a particular trade union;
- Conscientious objection; and
- Poverty and imprisonment.

Potential issues of importance include access to healthcare, 'postcode prescribing' and conscientious objection to abortion in relation to employment.

Conclusion

The Human Rights Act does not introduce any new rights that are not already covered by the Convention. Nevertheless it incorporates those rights directly into domestic law and makes them more accessible in British courts. While British Parliamentary sovereignty and tradition mean that any one Act of Parliament cannot bind a future Parliament, it is unlikely that the United Kingdom would unilaterally withdraw from the Convention or the Treaty underlying it. The Convention rights are likely to have a lasting effect on UK law. The above discussion of the potential areas of interest in medico-legal issues is limited at present. Nevertheless, the effects of the Human Rights Act on medical law are likely to be far-reaching within the next decade: see Table 2.3.

Keypoints

The Human Rights Act (HRA 1998) covers a wide range of issues in clinical practice and professional regulation. The HRA stresses the positive obligations of doctors and healthcare authorities. The HRA must be taken into account by British courts and will be influential in the development of common law.

Part 2

Consent, Confidentiality and Clinical Negligence

Chapter 3

Consent to treatment

Learning objectives

Core knowledge
- Legal requirement for consent
- Criteria for valid consent
- Definition of mental capacity
- Consent and children
- Principle of Necessity

Practical applications
- Assessment of capacity
- Obtaining valid consent
- Withholding of information
- Enduring Powers of Attorney (England & Wales)
- Welfare Attorneys and proxy decision-making (Scotland)

Background principles and case law
- Legal and ethical requirements for consent
- Consent in children and incompetent adults
- Compulsory detention and treatment in psychiatric patients
- Advance Statements
- Cases
  Gillick v. West Norfolk and Wisbech HA (1985)
  Re F (1990)
  Re T (1993)
  Re C (1994)
  Re MB (1997)
  Re AK (2001)

Consent is an essential requirement for medical and surgical treatment. Obtaining consent is an important clinical skill, which will have to be acquired during the pre-registration year as a House Officer. It needs good communication skills and a basic knowledge of what the law requires should be disclosed. Common complaints of patients when there are complications are that they would not have had the treatment if they had known the problems, and that they were not adequately informed about potential side-effects.

Children, psychiatric patients and the mentally incapacitated have particular problems regarding consent. The law in Scotland now permits proxy decision-making and may provide a model for similar changes to English law that, at the time of writing, are under consideration by the Westminster Parliament as part of the Mental Capacity Bill.

Introduction

The need for consent to treatment

Obtaining consent from a patient before treatment serves two purposes—one clinical, the other legal. The clinical purpose is to obtain the trust and co-operation of the patient. The fact that treatment is consensual is likely to contribute to its success.

Medical treatment can only lawfully be administered to a mentally capable adult with his or her consent.

Table 3.1. Inadequate consent may lead to claims in negligence, not trespass

> 'Once the patient is informed in broad terms of the nature of the procedure which is intended, and gives her consent, that consent is real, and the cause of the action on which to base a claim for failure to inform as to the risks and implications is negligence, not trespass.'
>
> Mr Justice Bristow in *Chatterton v Gerson* (1981)

Table 3.2. A competent patient has an absolute right to refuse consent

> 'A mentally competent patient has an absolute right to refuse consent to medical treatment for any reason, rational or irrational, or for no reason at all, even where that decision might lead to his death. The only situation in which it is lawful for the doctors to intervene is if it was believed that the adult patient lacked the capacity to decide and the treatment was in the patient's best interests.'
>
> Dame Elizabeth Butler-Sloss in *Re MB* (1997)

- Treatment of a mentally competent adult without consent constitutes trespass against the person. Hence, where a doctor treats a patient without their consent he or she risks criminal prosecution for assault and being sued for the tort of battery.
- Inadequate consent may lead to claims in negligence (Table 3.1).
- For consent to be legally valid, a patient must understand in broad terms the basic nature and purpose of the medical procedure. A doctor has a legal obligation to inform the patient. In English law a patient's apparent consent will be invalid if induced through fraud or misrepresentation as to the nature of the medical procedure.
- An adult patient of sound mind has an absolute legal right to refuse consent (Table 3.2).
- The right to refuse treatment also applies to the right of a pregnant woman to refuse a Caesarean section even though this may lead to harm, or even death, to herself or her unborn child following the case of *St George's Healthcare NHS Trust v S (1998)*.
- Where an adult patient is mentally incompetent, treatment may proceed under the English common law principle of necessity (see below).
- In English law at the time of writing, no one can give consent on behalf of a mentally competent adult, nor indeed for an adult who lacks mental capacity.
- The position in Scotland is different following the enactment of the Adults with Incapacity (Scotland) Act 2000. In Scottish law, patients may create powers of attorney to cover their health and welfare, which become operative when they become mentally incapable of making such decisions themselves. Moreover, the court may appoint a proxy decision-maker for the patient called, in Scotland, a Guardian. Proposals for similar legislation are being considered in England and Wales at the time of writing.
- Written consent provides documentary evidence of consent but is not proof of the adequacy of consent. The law is concerned with the quality of consent, which may be defective even in the face of a signed consent form.

Express consent

The validity and applicability of a patient's consent is more important than the form in which it is conveyed. Patients may express consent either orally or in writing. Written consent is particularly important to avoid subsequent misunderstandings between the doctor and patient and any others who are subsequently involved in the patient's care. Written consent is particularly important where:

1 The treatment is complex or involves significant risks.

2 Clinical care is not the primary purpose of the examination or investigation (e.g. when undertaken for insurance purposes).

3 There may be significant implications for the patient's employment, or social or personal life.

4 The treatment or investigation is part of a research programme.

5 It is a statutory requirement, e.g. in the case of infertility treatment.

Implied consent

The GMC warns of the dangers in assuming implied consent when, for example, it is assumed that a patient consents to be examined simply by lying down on an examination couch without an adequate explanation of what the doctor intends to do and why.

Reviewing and renewing consent

It is important that consent is up to date. The doctor primarily responsible, or a delegated member of the medical team, should review the patient's decision close to the time of treatment. This review is particularly important where:

1 Significant time has elapsed between obtaining consent and starting treatment.

2 There have been material changes in the patient's condition or the proposed treatment plan that might invalidate the patient's consent.

3 New and potentially relevant information has become available, e.g. concerning risks or other treatment options.

Consent to screening

Screening, particularly for genetic conditions, may have implications not only for the individual patient but also for others such as family members. The individual to be screened must be aware of the purpose of screening, the possibility of false positives and negatives, the uncertainties and risks attached to the screening process, significant medical, social or financial implications of the screening and any follow-up plans, including the availability of counselling and support services.

In the case of the screening of children and those without mental capacity, account should be taken of the guidance issued by bodies such as the Human Genetics Commission.

Consent to research

The conditions for obtaining consent in research projects from volunteers and patients are stringent, and rightly so. Before participating in research on competent patients or volunteers, it is important to ensure that the research is not contrary to the individuals' interests and that the participants understand that it is research and that the results are not predictable. Nevertheless, the GMC has not issued precise guidance on the issues surrounding non-therapeutic research on those who lack mental capacity. Instead, it refers to the relevant guidelines from bodies such as the Medical Research Council, the Association of the British Pharmaceutical Industry, the Nuffield Council on Bioethics and the World Health Organization.

Exceptions to the requirement of consent by the patient

There are certain legally recognized circumstances in which treatment may be given without the consent of the patient.

1 Necessary treatment in the case of mentally incapacitated adults.

2 Treatment of children under the age of 16 years.

3 Treatment of patients with mental disorder under the Mental Health Act 1983.

4 In Scotland, in cases where consent has been given by a Welfare Attorney, Court-appointed guardians, or a court (usually a Sheriff Court) on behalf of an incompetent adult.

Consent and mentally incapacitated adults

In English common law necessary medical treatment may be given without consent where the patient is mentally incapacitated, e.g. unconscious or demented. Such treatment must be in the patient's best medical interests following the case of *Re F* (1990), which was a case involving the sterilization of a mentally incompetent woman.

Lord Goff ruled:

'In making decisions about treatment, the doctor must act in accordance with a responsible and competent body of professional opinion, on the principles set down in *Bolam v Friern Hospital*. No doubt, in practice, a decision may involve others besides the doctor. It must surely be good practice to consult relatives and others who are concerned with the care of the patient. Sometimes, of course, consultation with a specialist or specialists will be required; and in others, especially where the decision involves more than a purely medical opinion, an inter-disciplinary team will in practice participate in the decision. It is very difficult, and would be unwise, for a court to do more than to stress that, for those who are involved in these important and sometimes difficult decisions, the overriding consideration is that they should act in the best interests of the person who suffers from the misfortune of being prevented by incapacity from deciding for himself what should be done to his own body, in his own best interests.'

Where a patient lacks mental capacity and is incapable of giving consent, treatment is justified under the common law principle of necessity (Table 3.3), as was explained by Lord Goff in the case of *Re F* (1990).

Consent and patients with mental disorder

According to Section 1(2) of the Mental Health Act 1983, mental disorder, means 'mental illness, arrested or incomplete development of mind, psychopathic disorder and any other disorder or disability of mind'. The presence of mental disorder does not of itself imply mental incapacity.

Table 3.3. Common Law Principle of Necessity

The conditions justifying treatment according to the Principle of Necessity are:
'Not only (1) must there be a necessity to act when it is not practicable to communicate with the assisted person, but also (2) the action taken must be such as a reasonable person would in all the circumstances take, acting in the best interests of the assisted person. . . . Action properly taken to preserve the life, health or well-being of the assisted person may well transcend such measures as surgical operations or substantial medical treatment and may extend to include such humdrum matters as routine medical or dental treatment, or even simple care such as dressing and undressing and putting to bed.' Lord Goff in *Re F* (1990)

Treatment under the Mental Health Act covers treatment of the underlying mental disorder and its consequences, but does not cover unrelated medical conditions. Hence nutritional support of patients with anorexia nervosa is justified if malnutrition or weight loss is a consequence of the mental disorder.

Additional safeguards for patients with mental disorder

There are additional safeguards for certain treatments under the Mental Health Act 1983.

Treatment limitation period

The administration of medicine beyond three months requires either the patient's consent or the approval of the Second Opinion Appointed Doctor (s.58)—except in case of emergency (s.62).

Specifically restricted treatments

There are certain treatments of mental disorder for which there are additional safeguards under the Mental Health Act. Live donor organ donation is illegal under the Human Organ Transplants Act 1989 without the donor's express consent. Consent is required for the treatment of children under the age of 16 years who are still subject to the authority of their parents or those standing in *loco parentis*.

Electroconvulsive therapy (ECT)

This either requires the patient's consent or, in the absence of consent, the approval of the Second Opinion Doctor (s.58) who must certify that ECT will alleviate or prevent deterioration in the patient's condition.

Neurosurgery

Surgical operations destroying brain tissue, and the surgical implantation of hormones to reduce the male sex drive, also require actual patient consent together with approval of the Second Opinion Doctor—(except for emergency treatment where treatment is regulated by s.62 of the Mental Health Act).

Non-therapeutic sterilization

This will normally require the sanction of the court, as in the case of *Re F* (1990).

In Scotland, those with parental responsibility cannot override the refusal of a competent child (Legal Capacity (Scotland) Act 1991, s.2.4).

Application to the court

Application to the Court is recommended by the GMC where the patient's capacity is in doubt, or where there is doubt about the patient's 'best interests'. A ruling ought to be sought for a non-therapeutic intervention in a mentally incapacitated adult, for example for contraceptive sterilization, organ donation, or withdrawal of life support from a PVS patient. The patient and his/her representatives should be informed of any decision to apply to the court and of their right to legal representation.

Patients may not demand treatments that are not clinically indicated, or are unnecessary or unduly hazardous. Patients cannot demand illegal treatment such as a prescription of illicit drugs, or mutilating surgery, e.g. female circumcision (Prohibition of Female Circumcision Act 1985).

Children and consent

Treatment of competent children (under the age of 16)

A child between the ages of 16 and 18 is presumed to have the same capacity to consent as an adult according to the Family Law Reform Act of 1969 s.8 (1). Under the age of 16 a child is presumed to be able to give consent if he or she is sufficiently intelligent and mature to be able to understand what the treatment involves. Such a child is regarded as 'Gillick competent'. (Table 3.4)

A child's capacity to give consent under the age of 16 years will depend upon the complexity of the procedures involved. A child may be able to under-

Table 3.4. The *Gillick* case

The Department of Health issued a circular to Health Authorities that advised that a doctor could give contraception advice and treatment to girls under the age of 16 if he was acting in good faith to protect the girl from the harmful effects of sexual intercourse. A doctor should normally proceed on the assumption that such help should normally be given with the knowledge and consent of the parents. However, the principle of confidentiality between doctor and patient also applied to those under 16 years of age, and in exceptional circumstances the doctor could prescribe contraceptives without parental consent if, in the judgement of the doctor, the child was capable of understanding what was involved and thus could give consent to the proposed treatment (i.e. prescription of contraceptives).

Mrs Victoria Gillick had five daughters under the age of 16 and sought assurance from her local Health Authority that they would not be given advice or treatment on contraception without her prior knowledge and agreement. When the authority refused she brought an action against the Health Authority, arguing that the advice was unlawful because:
● it amounted to causing or encouraging unlawful sexual intercourse in a girl under 16 contrary to ss. 6 and 28 of the Sexual Offences Act 1956 and
● it was inconsistent with parental rights.
The judge at first instance refused her application, but the Court of Appeal unanimously allowed her appeal. The Department of Health then appealed to the House of Lords, who overturned the decision of the Court of Appeal by a 3 to 2 majority.

Gillick v West Norfolk and Wisbech Health Authority
(1985)

stand and consent to the setting of a broken arm but unable to understand the full implications of a bone marrow transplant.

Lord Scarman, giving the leading judgment in the Gillick case, stated:

'Save where statute otherwise provides, a minor's capacity to make his or her own decision depends upon the minor having sufficient understanding and intelligence to make the decision and is not to be determined by references to any judicially fixed age limit. . . . I would hold that as a matter of law the parental right to determine whether or not their minor child below the age of 16 will have medical treatment terminates if and when the child achieves a sufficient understanding and intelligence to enable him or her to understand what is proposed.'

Where a child is unable to consent and is thereby regarded at law as incompetent to make a decision regarding medical treatment, the power to consent rests with the parents, or others with parental responsibility, such as a local authority if the child is in care. The court affirmed that:

'Until the child achieves the capacity to consent, the parental right to make the decision continues save only in exceptional circumstances.'

Situations may arise where the child's life is threatened or there is risk of serious permanent harm. In the case of *Re R* (1991) the refusal by a 15-year-old of her anti-psychotic medication was overruled by the court. At the subsequent Court of Appeal ruling it was confirmed that the court, acting in a wardship capacity, could overrule the decisions of a 'Gillick competent' child as well as the child's parents or guardians.

Lord Donaldson (as Master of the Rolls, the senior judge of the Court of Appeal) in *Re R* stated that:

'In a case in which the "Gillick competent" child refuses treatment, but the parents consent, that consent enables treatment to be undertaken lawfully, but in no way determines that the child shall be so treated. In a case in which the positions are reversed, it is the child's consent which is the enabling factor and again the parents' refusal of consent is not determinative.'

While a child's consent to treatment may be valid in law, the child's refusal is not necessarily valid. Hence a parent or guardian may give consent notwithstanding a child's refusal. Some of Lord Donaldson's conclusions in the case of *Re R* concerning the rights and responsibilities of doctors, parents and the courts in relation to the decisions of a 'Gillick competent' child are outlined in Table 3.5.

In Scotland, those with parental responsibility cannot override the refusal of a competent child (Legal Capacity (Scotland) Act 1991 s.2.4), and the

Table 3.5. Rights and responsibilities of doctors, parents and the courts in relation to the 'Gillick competent' child

(1) No doctor can be required to treat a child, whether by the court in the exercise of its wardship jurisdiction, by the parents, by the child or anyone else. The decision whether to treat is dependent upon an exercise of his own professional judgment, subject only to the threshold requirement that, save in exceptional cases, usually of emergency, he has the consent of someone who has authority to give that consent. In forming that judgment the views and wishes of the child are a factor whose importance increases with the increase in the child's intelligence and understanding.
(2) There can be concurrent powers to consent. If more than one body or person has a power to consent, only a failure to, or refusal of, consent by all having that power will create a veto.
(3) A 'Gillick competent' child or one over the age of 16 will have a power to consent, but this will be concurrent with that of a parent or guardian.
(4) 'Gillick competence' is a developmental concept and will not be lost or acquired on a day-to-day or week-to-week basis. In the case of mental disability, that disability must also be taken into account, particularly where it is fluctuating in its effect.
(5) The court in the exercise of its wardship or statutory jurisdiction has power to override the decisions of a 'Gillick competent' child as much as those of parents or guardians.

Lord Donaldson in *Re R (a minor) (wardship: medical treatment)* (1991)

Scottish Act refers to 'procedures', not just 'treatment', as the English 1969 Act does, and is thus wider in scope.

Consent to treatment for those between 16 and 18 years

The common law position relating to 'Gillick competence' applies to those up to 16 years of age. The Family Law Reform Act of 1969, s.8(1), applies to medical treatment of those aged 16 to 18 years (Table 3.6).

In the case of *Re W* (1993) it was recognized that the refusal of a 16-year-old could be overridden.

W was a girl of 16 suffering from anorexia nervosa and was refusing treatment. Lord Donaldson

Table 3.6. Consent of children who have reached the age of 16 years

> 8.(1)The consent of a minor who has attained the age of 16 years to any surgical, medical or dental treatment which, in the absence of consent, would constitute a trespass to his person, shall be as effective as it would be if he were of full age; and where a minor has by virtue of this section given an effective consent to any treatment it shall not be necessary to obtain any consent for it from his parent or guardian.
>
> Family Law Reform Act 1969 s.8(1)

Table 3.7. The case of C: Refusal of amputation

> C was a 68-year-old paranoid schizophrenic in Broadmoor who had developed a gangrenous foot. A below-knee amputation was deemed necessary to prevent the spread of gangrene. The patient, who believed that he was an internationally recognized doctor, applied for, and was granted, an injunction preventing amputation at that time and at any future date.
>
> Re C (Adult: Refusal of treatment) 1994

in the Court of Appeal did not consider that s.8 related to refusal of treatment in the same way it did with consent to treatment and that the court had wide powers under wardship, notwithstanding s.8.

Treatment of incompetent minors

Under the Children Act 1989, the parent with 'parental responsibility' can give consent unless that responsibility is removed or restricted (s.33(3) and (4)). Others such as teachers and childminders may, as a matter of fact, have the power to consent and are given it in the words of s.3 (5).

> 'A person who does not have parental responsibility for a particular child, but has care of the child' may 'do what is reasonable in all the circumstances of the case for the purpose of safeguarding and promoting the child's welfare'.

In the words of Lord Donaldson (Master of the Rolls) in the case of *Re C* (1990):

> 'The origin of the wardship jurisdiction is the duty of the Crown to protect its subjects and particularly children, who are the generations of the future. It is exercised by the courts on behalf of the Crown . . . The machinery for its exercise is an application to make the child a ward of court. Thereafter, the court is entitled and bound in appropriate cases to make decisions in the interests of the child which override the rights of its parents. Furthermore, the court is entitled, and bound in appropriate cases, to make orders affecting third parties which the parents could not themselves have made.'

Where a person with parental responsibility reasonably refuses treatment for a child under the age of 16 years who lacks capacity, the court may override that decision. In an emergency, the GMC recognizes that a doctor may provide necessary treatment in the face of such a refusal in the child's best medical interests.

Criteria for valid consent to treatment

Mental capacity

Mental capacity is ultimately a legal issue for the courts to decide, even though doctors and others may assist the court in arriving at a decision. There are legal presumptions that a patient has capacity (presumption of capacity) and that a state of competence, or incompetence, is permanent (presumption of continuance) unless the contrary can be shown.

A patient is deemed competent if, at the material time that consent is given, he is capable of understanding what is involved, including the procedure itself, the consequences of treatment and the consequences of not receiving treatment.

The High Court set criteria for adult mental capacity in the case of *Re C* (1994) (Table 3.7).

Mr Justice Thorpe considered the relevant question in determining C's mental capacity was whether 'Mr C's capacity is so reduced by his chronic mental illness that he does not sufficiently understand the nature, purpose and effects of the proffered amputation.' Dr Eastman, a forensic psychiatrist and expert witness in the case, suggested a three-stage test of 'capacity' that was accepted by the court. This has become known as the 'C test'.

The High Court held that an adult has capacity to consent (or refuse consent) to medical treatment if he or she can:

1 Understand and retain the information relevant to the decision in question;

2 Believe that information; and

3 Weigh that information and arrive at a choice.

According to the Master of the Rolls, Lord Donaldson, in the case of *Re T* (1993), it is important that doctors give careful consideration to the patient's mental capacity in the face of a refusal of treatment. He proposed a functional definition of capacity depending on the gravity of the decision in question.

'What matters is that the doctors consider whether at that time he had a capacity which was commensurate with the gravity of the decision; the graver the decision the greater the capacity required. If the patient had the requisite capacity, they are bound by his decision. If not, they are free to treat him in what they believe to be his best interests.'

In the case of *Re MB (an adult: medical treatment)* (1997) Dame Elizabeth Butler-Sloss propounded guidelines for deciding issues of capacity, including decisions made when the patient is pregnant (Table 3.8).

The guidelines used for deciding capacity were:

1 There is a rebuttable presumption of mental capacity. The graver the decision the greater the degree of competence required.

2 A patient with capacity has a right to make a decision that is rational, or irrational, or for no reason at all, even when the consequence may be death (or the death of an unborn child if the woman is pregnant).

3 Panic, irrationality or indecisiveness do not of themselves constitute incompetence, although may provide evidence of incompetence.

4 A patient lacks capacity if unable to understand the nature and need for treatment and to weigh it in the balance.

5 Capacity may be temporarily impaired by such factors as confusion, panic, shock or fatigue.

Table 3.8. The case of Miss MB: refusal of Caesarean section

Miss MB had often objected to needles during her pregnancy. When she was 40 weeks pregnant it was found that the foetus was in a breech position. Although there was an estimated 50% chance that the foetus would be harmed unless delivered by Caesarean section, Miss MB was in no personal danger. Unfortunately Miss MB's needle phobia made Caesarean section all but impossible. Whilst she agreed in principle to the operation, her fears led to panic and she refused surgery. The Health Authority applied for a declaration that it would be lawful to use reasonable force to insert a needle so that surgery could proceed. There was an appeal against the decision by Mr Justice Hollis that Miss MB lacked the capacity to consent or refuse treatment. At appeal it was held that MB was mentally incapacitated by virtue of her needle phobia.

Re MB (an adult: medical treatment) (1997)

Table 3.9. The Mental Health Code of Practice (1990) for determining mental competence

In order to have capacity a patient must be able to:

1. Understand what is meant by medical treatment, that it is needed and why it is needed.

2. Understand in broad terms the nature of the treatment that is proposed.

3. Understand the risks attached to the treatment as well as the benefits of it.

4. Understand what will happen if the treatment does not take place.

5. Have the capacity to make a choice.

In addition the Code suggested that:

(1) The assessment of capacity should be made with a specific proposal of treatment in mind.

(2) The assessment needs to be made at the time that the treatment is proposed. In many cases lucidity and mental disorder will not be constant.

(3) There should be full recording of capacity assessments in the patient's notes.

6 Panic induced by fear needs to be treated with caution when reviewing the evidence.

The Mental Health Act Code of Practice (1990) sets out series of criteria to be used in determining competence (Table 3.9).

Table 3.10. The *Sidaway* case

In the case of *Sidaway*, the plaintiff required an operation on a cervical vertebra to alleviate pain. The operation carried a 2% risk of damage to a nerve root and a 1% risk of damage to the spinal cord itself. In the event Mrs Sidaway suffered serious post-operative disability. The operation had been performed competently, but the patient had not been warned of the risk of the spinal injury that she had unfortunately sustained, though the less serious risk of nerve root damage had been mentioned.

In the House of Lords, Lord Bridge outlined the central issue:

'The important question which this appeal raises is whether the law imposes any, and if so what, different criterion as the measure of the medical man's duty of care to his patient when giving evidence with respect to a proposed course of treatment. It is clearly right to recognise that a conscious adult of sound mind is entitled to decide for himself whether or not he will submit to a particular course of treatment proposed by the doctor, most significantly surgical treatment under general anaesthesia.'

Sidaway v Bethlem Royal Hospital Governors and others (1985)

Adequacy of information

Disclosure of information

The extent of the duty to disclose information to patients was comprehensively stated in *Sidaway* (1985) (Table 3.10).

In the case of *Sidaway*, it was held by Lord Bridge that:

'In a case where, as here, no expert witness in the relevant medical field condemns the non-disclosure as being in conflict with accepted and responsible medical practice, I am of the opinion that the judge might in certain circumstances come to the conclusion that disclosure of a particular risk was so obviously necessary to an informed choice on the part of the patient that no reasonably prudent medical man would fail to make it.'

and that:

'When questioned specifically by a patient of apparently sound mind about the risk involved in a particular treatment proposed, the doctor's duty is to answer both truthfully and as fully as the questioner requires.'

Withholding information

Whether a particular risk is withheld or disclosed remains primarily a clinical matter, but the law nevertheless retains the power to intervene and to decide what is a reasonable degree of disclosure. However, as *Sidaway* makes clear, it will be a fairly obvious failure to disclose or a failure to disclose when asked (save where disclosure might harm the patient) that will invite the intervention of the court.

In *Sidaway* Lord Scarman said:

'The profession . . . should not be judge in its own cause; or, less emotively but more correctly, the courts should not allow medical opinion as to what is best for the patient to override the patient's right to decide for himself whether he will submit to the treatment offered him.'

and further:

'My conclusion as to the law is therefore this. To the extent that I have indicated, I think that English law must recognise a duty of the doctor to warn his patient of risk inherent in the treatment which he is proposing, and especially so if the treatment be surgery. The critical limitation is that the duty is confined to material risk. The test of materiality is whether in the circumstances of the particular case, the court is satisfied that a reasonable person in the patient's position would be likely to attach significance to the risk. Even if the risk be material, the doctor will not be liable if on a reasonable assessment of his patient's condition he takes the view that a warning would be detrimental to his patient's health.'

GMC guidelines on obtaining consent for treatment

In 1998 the GMC published detailed guidelines on

obtaining consent to treatment, entitled *Seeking patient's consent: the ethical considerations.*

According to the GMC, withholding information from a patient may be justified if it is felt that it would cause the patient serious harm to be given it. However, by 'serious harm' the GMC did not merely mean that the patient would be upset or decide to refuse treatment. Where a patient insists that they do not wish to know in detail about their condition and treatment, basic information must still be provided. Where a relative insists on information being withheld, the views of the patient ought to be sought and the relevant information ought not to be withheld unless it is felt it would cause the patient serious harm. A record should be kept of any information that is withheld and of the reason for non-disclosure. Doctors must be prepared to defend such non-disclosures.

The amount of information given to a patient regarding the treatment options and outlook will depend upon the nature of the condition and the complexity of the treatment. Such information should normally include the risks of the treatment or procedure, and the likely diagnosis and prognosis, including the likely outcome if the condition is left untreated. The purpose of the treatment should be discussed, including what the patient may experience and the common and any serious possible side-effects, including any changes in lifestyle that may be caused. Doctors should also inform patients of their right to a second opinion, or to withdraw from treatment and, in the case of private practice, any charges or costs that may be incurred. The information should be tailored to the individual patient's needs. Patients' views should not be assumed, and any special concerns they may have about any risks involved, including those to which they would attach particular importance, should be discussed.

The GMC warns doctors not to go beyond the scope of the authority given by the patient, except in an emergency. This may be particularly relevant where the treatment is to be given in stages or when different doctors or other health care workers provide particular elements of investigation or treatment, or where there is uncertainty over the diagnosis or appropriate treatment or when the patient may be unable to participate in decision-making. In such instances there 'should be clear agreement whether the patient consents to all or only parts of the proposed plan of investigation or treatment, and whether further consent will have to be sought at a later stage'. Furthermore, where there is a possibility of additional problems arising during a procedure when the patient is unconscious (e.g. during general anaesthesia), the patient should be asked if there are any procedures to which they would object or wish to give further thought to before proceeding.

If, in exceptional circumstances, the doctor was to treat an unconscious patient in a way that fell outside the scope of the consent, the decision could be challenged in the courts, by the employing authority, or even by the GMC. The onus now lies with the doctor to justify his actions. Furthermore, any unauthorized treatment given to an unconscious patient without consent ought to be disclosed to the patient as soon as they have sufficiently recovered to understand what has happened to them.

Questions raised by the patient should be answered honestly and as far as the patient wishes, including whether the risks and benefits of treatment are affected by the choice of institution or doctor providing the care.

Information should be presented to patients in a way and at a time that the patient is best able to understand and retain it. Obtaining consent involves a continuing dialogue with the patient, and may involve, where appropriate and practicable, written, visual and other aids. The patient may wish to consult relatives or friends, and might find making tape-recordings of conversations useful.

Patients should be given distressing information in a considerate way, and provided with information about counselling services and patient support groups as appropriate. Time should be allowed for due consideration of the risks and benefits of treatment, and, where time elapses between the giving of consent and the start of treatment, the patient should review the decision with the person providing the treatment.

The GMC makes it clear that the primary responsibility for obtaining consent rests with the doctor providing the treatment or undertaking an investigation. This task may only be delegated to someone who is suitably trained and has sufficient practical knowledge and is aware of the risks involved.

Doctrine of 'informed consent' and the 'prudent patient test'

Contrary to popular belief, there is no doctrine of 'informed consent' in English law (as to some degree there is in America).

The so-called 'prudent patient test' recognizes the right of self-determination of the patient. It sets the standard as to what information is required for valid consent according to what the reasonable or prudent patient would wish to know under the circumstances. However, Lord Bridge, in *Sidaway*, rejected the 'prudent patient' test on three counts:

1 It gives insufficient weight to the doctor–patient relationship. A number of factors need to be taken into account in forming the doctor's clinical judgement, not only in relation to the diagnosis and likely outcome and the risks and benefits of treatment (and non-treatment), but also in relation to the best way to inform the patient so that a well-considered and balanced decision can be made. It is clearly impossible to educate the patient to his own standard of medical knowledge.

2 It would be unreasonable in any clinical negligence claim to restrict expert medical opinion to the primary medical factors and to deny the court the benefit of medical opinion and practice on the issue of disclosure.

3 The objective test required according to the 'prudent patient' criterion is so imprecise as to be meaningless. Hence, if it is left to an individual judge to decide what 'a reasonable person in the patient's position' would consider a significant risk, the outcome of litigation is likely to become wholly unpredictable.

The GMC has made it clear that 'It is for the patient, not the doctor, to decide on "what is in the patient's own best interest"'. The GMC stresses that pressure should not be placed on patients to accept a doctor's advice. Patients detained under the Mental Health Act or by police or immigration

Table 3.11. The case of Miss T: refusal of a blood transfusion

Miss T was 34 weeks pregnant and was rushed to hospital after a road traffic accident. Her mother was a Jehovah's Witness, although T was not. Following admission to hospital and discussions with her mother, T declared that she shared some of the beliefs of Jehovah's Witnesses, including the view that blood transfusion was a sin. She therefore signed a form refusing blood transfusion. As a result of the car accident, she went into premature labour. Her condition deteriorated, and a Caesarean Section became necessary. She was placed on a ventilator and given paralysing drugs. It was decided that a transfusion would not be unlawful in the absence of consent. An appeal was made against the decision and Lord Donaldson (Master of the Rolls) authorized transfusion.
Re T (Adult: Refusal of Treatment) (1993)

services or those in prison are particularly vulnerable and should be reminded of their rights to decline treatment, where appropriate.

Freedom from coercion or undue pressure

Consent must be freely given without undue coercion or pressure following *Re T* (1993) (Table 3.11).

In addition to deciding the question of undue influence or coercion, the case of *Re T* is a source of several useful statements concerning consent, especially for life-saving treatment.

- Every adult has the right to accept or refuse treatment, even if refusal would lead to permanent injury or death. Any such refusal can be for reasons that are rational or irrational, unknown or even not in existence. However, there is a strong public interest in the preservation of life. Therefore the presumption that all adults have capacity is rebuttable.
- Lack of capacity may be long-standing, e.g. due to retarded development, or temporary, due to unconsciousness, pain, shock or the effects of drugs.
- Where the patient lacks capacity, doctors have a duty to treat a patient in that patient's best interests.
- Doctors may be faced with situations of reduced capacity. What matters is whether at the time the

patient's capacity was reduced below the level needed to refuse treatment, bearing in mind that the refusal of some treatment may involve a risk to life or of irreparable damage to health. The degree of capacity needed to make a serious decision is greater than for a trivial one.

- Doctors in deciding capacity must be aware of the possibility of undue influence that might vitiate consent.
- Doctors will need to consider the precise scope of the refusal, and whether it was meant to cover the situation actually encountered. A refusal may be vitiated if it rests on a false assumption of the circumstances.
- Patients may need to be clearly reminded of the consequences of a refusal, especially a refusal of life-saving treatment.
- The assistance of the court should be sought in cases of doubt.

Capacity to establish an enduring power of attorney

The Enduring Powers of Attorney Act 1985 allows individuals to make arrangements for an attorney to deal with their assets and affairs after they have become incapacitated. Hence, an enduring power of attorney is one that 'endures', or continues, after the donor has become mentally incapacitated, provided it has been registered with the Office of the Court of Protection of the High Court.

The conditions for the creation of an enduring Power of Attorney are set out in the 1985 Act and commented upon in the cases *Re K* and *Re F*. The person creating the Power of Attorney must understand:

1 If such be the terms of the power, that the attorney will be able to assume complete authority over the donor's affairs;

2 If such be the terms of the power, that the attorney will be able to do anything with the donor's property that the donor could have done;

3 That the authority will continue if the donor should be, or should become, mentally incapable; and

4 That if he or she should be or should become mentally incapable, the power will be irrevocable

without the need for any confirmation of the Court of Protection.

Proxy decision-making

In *Re F* (1990) it was held that in English Law there was no procedure whereby a substitute or proxy can be appointed with the power to consent to treatment on behalf of a mentally incompetent adult. However, the High Court has the jurisdiction to make a declaration (which is governed by the Civil Procedure Rules), as to whether or not a given act is lawful. Nevertheless, declaratory relief by the High Court does not bind anyone not party to the legal case, and 'will not alter the legal status of the proposed conduct', as the court re-affirmed in *Airedale NHS Trust v Bland* (1993), the well-known case of Tony Bland, the Hillsborough Stadium victim.

In Scotland, however, the Adults with Incapacity (Scotland) Act 2000 permits proxy—decision-making by Welfare Attorneys and Court-Appointed Managers.

Adults with incapacity (Scotland) Act 2000

This Act was passed by the Scottish Parliament and allows proxy decision-making by Welfare Attorneys, appointed by the patient, and court-appointed managers called 'guardians'.

Part I of the Act includes a general authority to act reasonably on behalf of an incapacitated adult. The principle is expressed in s.1(2) and (3):

1 There shall be no intervention in the affairs of an adult unless the person responsible for authorizing or effecting the intervention is satisfied that the intervention will benefit the adult and that such benefit cannot reasonably be achieved without the intervention.

2 Where it is determined that an intervention as mentioned in sub-section (1) is to be made, such intervention shall be the least restrictive option in relation to the freedom of the adult, consistent with the purpose of the intervention.

In deciding what intervention is to be made, account must be taken of the wishes of the adult, in so far as they can be ascertained, and the views of the nearest relative and primary carer, as well as those of any guardian, welfare attorney or other person whom the Sheriff has directed ought to be consulted.

Part 5 of the Act concerns the medical treatment of the incapacitated adult. S.47(2) allows 'the medical practitioner primarily responsible for the medical treatment of the adult . . . authority to do what is reasonable in the circumstances, in relation to the medical treatment, to safeguard or promote the physical or mental health of the adult'.

However, the general authority to treat reasonably under s.47(2) does not apply 'where a guardian or a welfare attorney has been appointed'.

Indeed, where there is a disagreement regarding the treatment of an incapable adult between the doctor and welfare attorney, the medical practitioner 'shall request the Mental Welfare Commission to nominate a medical practitioner (the "nominated medical practitioner") from the list established and maintained by them under subsection (9) to give an opinion as to the medical treatment proposed'.

Where the nominated medical practitioner certifies that, in his opinion, having regard to all the circumstances and having consulted the guardian, welfare attorney or other authorized person, that the treatment may be given, then it may proceed. However, where the nominated doctor agrees with the proxy that the treatment should be withdrawn or withheld, then it can only be given if the doctor primarily responsible for the patient has been granted permission to proceed by the Court of Session (the Scottish equivalent of the English High Court).

Advance statements and 'best interests'

According to the GMC guidelines, doctors 'must respect any refusal of treatment given when the patient was competent, provided the decision in the Advance Statement is clearly applicable to the present circumstances, and there is no reason to believe that the patient has changed his/her mind. Where

an Advance Statement of this kind is not available, the patient's known wishes should be taken into account—on the "best interests" principle'. The 'best interests' of the patient are defined according to the following criteria:

1 Options for treatment or investigation that are clinically indicated;

2 The patient's previously expressed preferences, including an Advance Statement;

3 The patient's known background, and cultural, religious and employment considerations;

4 Views concerning preferences obtained from a third party; and

5 The option that least restricts the patient's future choices.

Doctors are qualified to make decisions based upon the clinical best interests of the patient, and any non-clinical criteria must come ultimately from the patient. Moreover, the doctor must be sure that the patient's *present* wishes are respected, and while an Advance Statement is useful evidentially, caution must be exercised that it does not override the patient's current wishes, which may well have changed, or fail to take into account some factor not envisaged by the Advance Statement.

The current state of the law regarding Advance Statements was stated by Mr Justice Hughes in the case of *Re AK* (2001), and provides very useful practical as well as legal guidance on the subject. The judge said:

'It is clearly the law that the doctors are not entitled so to act if it is known that the patient, provided he was of sound mind and full capacity, has let it be known that he does not consent and that such treatment is against his wishes. To this extent an advanced indication of the wishes of a patient of full capacity and sound mind are effective. Care will of course have to be taken to ensure that such anticipatory declarations of wishes still represent the wishes of the patient. Care must be taken to investigate how long ago the expression of wishes was made. Care must be taken to investigate with what knowledge the expression of wishes was made. All the circumstances in which the expression of wishes was given will of course have to be investigated. In the present case the expressions of AK's decision are recent and made not on any hypothetical basis but in the fullest possible knowledge of impending reality.'

Conclusion

The rights and duties of the doctor are co-relative to those of the competent adult patient both ethically and legally. The physician has no separate or independent right over the mentally capable patient, and can treat only in so far as the patient gives him permission. Treatment without proper consent constitutes trespass against the person, and the doctor may risk prosecution for assault or even battery.

Chapter 4

Confidentiality

Introduction

Confidentiality is central to the relationship between doctors and patients, and its ethical significance was recognized in the Hippocratic Oath. Without assurances about confidentiality, patients would be reluctant to give information about themselves that is necessary for their medical care. Personal information about patients should not normally be divulged without the patient's consent (or that of a parent or guardian in the case of children) unless the disclosure can be justified on the basis of preventing harm to the patient or others.

Table 4.1 Duty of confidentiality

'. . . a duty of confidence arises when confidential information comes to the knowledge of a person (the confidant) in circumstances where he has notice, or is held to have agreed, that the information is confidential, with the effect that it would be just in all circumstances that he should be precluded from disclosing the information to others'.
Lord Goff in *Attorney-General v Guardian Newspapers Ltd (no.2)* (1990)

Confidentiality is regulated by GMC Guidelines and by certain Acts of Parliament such as the Access to Medical Reports Act 1988, the Access to Health Records Act 1990, the Data Protection Act 1998 and the Human Rights Act 1998.

Lord Goff defined the duty of confidentiality in common law in the famous *Spycatcher* trial (Table 4.1).

Patients' right to confidentiality

The patient's right of confidentiality is protected by the common law, statutes, disciplinary codes and policies and contracts of employment of healthcare staff.

The Human Rights Act entails a positive legal duty to respect confidentiality. Article 8 states:

'Everyone has a right to respect for his private and family life, his home and his correspondence.'

However, Article 8 allows for restriction of this right where it is necessary:

'in the interests of national security, public safety or the economic well-being of the country, the prevention of disorder or crime, for the protection of health or morals, or for the protection of the rights and freedoms of others.'

According to the GMC's guidelines 'patients have a right to information about any condition or disease from which they are suffering. This should be presented in a manner easy to follow and use, and include information about the diagnosis, prognosis, treatment options, outcomes of treatment, common and/or serious side-effects of treatment, a likely time-scale of treatment and costs where relevant.' (*Confidentiality. Protecting and providing information*, GMC, 2000).

Nevertheless, while patients have a right to information about their condition and treatment, they also have a right not to be given detailed information, should they so choose. The GMC continues:

'You should always give patients basic information about treatment you propose to provide, but you should respect the wishes of any patient who asks you not to give them detailed information. This places a considerable onus upon health professionals.'

The Freedom of Information Act 2000

From 1 January 2005, the Freedom of Information Act 2000 will give a general statutory right of access to all types of recorded information held by public authorities. A member of the public will be able to access information held by various public authorities, including Parliament, government departments, local authorities, health trusts, doctors' surgeries and many other organizations.

Disclosure of personal information

The GMC recognizes that there are circumstances in which it is reasonable to disclose, or share, information with others for the direct or indirect benefit of the patient:

● Amongst other members of the healthcare professions involved in the treatment and care of the patient, e.g. in correspondence between GPs and Consultants.

● Between members of the healthcare team.

● For purposes of education, research, epidemiology, public health, surveillance, audit, administration and planning.

Disclosure should be in accord with the following principles:

● Seek the patient's consent wherever possible, whether or not individual patients can be identified from the disclosure.

● Disclosures should be kept to a minimum.

● Anonymized data should be used where possible.

Seeking the patient's consent to disclosure

Express consent (orally or in writing) ought to be obtained when the patient may be affected by the disclosure of information, e.g. in relation to employment or insurance.

● Where the patient is unlikely to be personally affected by the disclosure of information, the patient should still be told that their records may be revealed to others, of the purpose of the disclosure, and of their right to object to the release of information.

● Those having access to such information are also under a duty of confidentiality.

● Disclosures may be made in the public interest without the consent of the patient where the benefits likely to arise from disclosure outweigh the possible harm to the patient and the trust implicit in the doctor–patient relationship.

● It will be for the courts to decide what is in the 'public interest', although the GMC has made it clear that it may also require justification for the release of information without the patient's consent.

Disclosures that indirectly benefit patients

Disclosure of information about patients may be important for:
- Public health and healthcare planning
- Drug safety, e.g. the yellow card scheme run by the Committee on the Safety of Medicines
- Service provision, e.g. Cancer Registries
- Confidential enquiries, e.g. those into maternal mortality and perioperative mortality
- Epidemiological surveys, e.g. into communicable diseases.

The GMC has stated that automatic transfer of personal data to a registry is unacceptable (but see below for a qualification of this stance). It says:

> 'The automatic transfer of personal information to a registry, whether by electronic or other means, before informing the patient that information will be passed on, is unacceptable save in the most exceptional circumstances. These would be where a court has already decided that there is such an overwhelming public interest in the disclosure of information to a registry that patients' rights to confidentiality are overridden; or where you are willing and able to justify the disclosure, potentially before a court or to the GMC, on the same grounds.'

Where named or identifiable information is given to a cancer registry, oral or written consent from the patient should be obtained, in keeping with GMC guidelines, the Data Protection Act 1998, the Human Rights Act 1998 and the common law.

Where medical research uses identifiable information or samples and it is not practicable to contact patients to obtain consent, the research ethics committee should be notified so that it can consider whether the likely research benefits outweigh the loss of confidentiality. However, in the event of a claim for breach of confidentiality it would be for the court to decide if the public interest had been served.

Disclosures where the doctor has dual responsibility

Situations may arise when a doctor has contractual obligations to third parties, for example where doctors work in occupational health services, insurance companies, agencies assessing claims or benefits or when working as police surgeons, in the armed forces, or in the prison service.

When asked to provide a report about a patient, the doctor must be satisfied that:
- The patient has been informed of the nature and purpose of the examination and report and that relevant information cannot be withheld.
- The patient, or someone authorized to act on their behalf, has provided written consent.
- Only relevant information has been disclosed.

The Access to Medical Reports Act 1988 entitles a patient to see written reports about them before they are disclosed, in some circumstances. In all cases the doctor should check if the patients wish to see their reports.

Disclosures to protect the patient or others from harm

Disclosure to prevent harm to others may arise, for example, where the patient is a doctor and is placing other patients at risk as a result of illness, e.g. of a serious infectious disease. A list of notifiable communicable diseases is given in Table 4.2. Category A infections must be notified to the local authority.
- Where disclosure may assist in the detection or prevention of serious crime. Serious crimes will include offences against the person where there is a risk of death or serious harm or child abuse.
- Where a patient continues to drive against medical advice.

According to the GMC:

> 'In such circumstances you should disclose relevant information to the medical adviser of the Driver and Vehicle Licensing Agency without delay.'

Advice to doctors from the GMC as to informing the DVLA if the patient refuses is shown in Table 4.3.

Table 4.2 Notifiable infectious diseases under the Public Health (Control of Diseases) Act 1984 and the Public Health (Infectious Diseases) Regulations 1988

Category A infections: Cholera, plague, relapsing fever, smallpox, typhus.

Category B infections: Acute encephalitis, acute poliomyelitis, meningitis (viral or bacterial), meningococcccal septicaemia, anthrax, diphtheria, dysentery, food poisoning, paratyphoid fever, typhoid fever, typhus, viral hepatitis, leprosy, leptospirosis, measles, mumps, rubella, whooping cough, malaria, tetanus, yellow fever, ophthalmia neonatorum, scarlet fever, tuberculosis, rabies, viral haemorrhagic fevers, Lassa fever, Marburg disease.

Note: there are a number of diseases that are not notifiable, including Chicken pox, Legionnaires' Disease, VTEC (verocytotoxin, producing *Escherichia coli* O157), vCJD and SARS (Severe Acute Respiratory Syndrome) and certain sexually transmitted diseases.

Disclosures after a patient's death

While there is still a general obligation to maintain confidentiality after a patient dies, there are a number of circumstances justifying release of information about patients who have died.

• In response to a Coroner or Procurator Fiscal (in Scotland).

• As part of a National Confidential Enquiry, audit, research or public health surveillance. Publication of anonymized data would be unlikely to be improper in these contexts.

• Death certification.

The Data Protection Act 1990 only covers the records of living patients. Claims arising in relation to those who have died are set out in the Access to Health Records Act 1990 or Access to Health Records (Northern Ireland) Order 1992. Such claims may arise in relation to insurance matters after death, and information should be released in accord with these legal provisions or with the authorization of those lawfully entitled to deal with the patient's estate.

Disclosure in relation to judicial or statutory proceedings

There may be a statutory requirement to notify

Table 4.3 Advice of the GMC regarding disclosure of information about patients to the Driver and Vehicle Licensing Agency (DVLA)

1. The DVLA is legally responsible for deciding if a person is medically unfit to drive. They need to know when driving licence holders have a condition which may, now or in the future, affect their safety as a driver.
2. Therefore, where patients have such conditions, you should:
   a. Make sure that the patients understand that the condition may impair their ability to drive. If a patient is incapable of understanding this advice, for example because of dementia, you should inform the DVLA immediately.
   b. Explain to patients that they have a legal duty to inform the DVLA about the condition.
3. If the patients refuse to accept the diagnosis or the effect of the condition on their ability to drive, you can suggest that the patients seek a second opinion, and make appropriate arrangements for the patients to do so. You should advise patients not to drive until the second opinion has been obtained.
4. If patients continue to drive when they are not fit to do so, you should make every reasonable effort to persuade them to stop. This may include telling their next of kin.
5. If you do not manage to persuade patients to stop driving, or you are given or find evidence that a patient is continuing to drive contrary to advice, you should disclose relevant medical information immediately, in confidence, to the medical adviser at DVLA.
6. Before giving information to the DVLA you should inform the patient of your decision to do so. Once the DVLA has been informed, you should also write to the patient, to confirm that a disclosure has been made.

Confidentiality: Protecting and Providing Information.
GMC. 2000

particular conditions such as infectious diseases or operations such as abortion.

1 Abortion regulations 1991 (SI 1991/499)

This relates to limited disclosure by the Chief Medical Officer of information that may be of concern to the DPP.

2 Public Health (Infectious Diseases) Regulations 1988 (SI 1988/1546)

This concerns a list of contagious diseases that must be notified to the appropriate authority.

3 National Health Service (Venereal Diseases) Regulations 1974 (SI 1974/29)

Information must be disclosed by order of a judge or the presiding officer of a court, but should not be disclosed to a solicitor or police officer without the express consent of the patient unless it be to prevent harm to the patient or others or to prevent serious crime.

Information may also be disclosed to an official request from a statutory regulatory body such as the General Medical or Dental Council.

S.9 of the Police and Criminal Evidence Act 1984 allows special access to 'excluded material', which includes 'human tissue or tissue fluid which has been taken for the purposes of diagnosis or medical treatment and which a person holds in confidence'. Ss.11 and 12 also allow access to personal medical records in the course of criminal investigations.

Provisions for sexually transmitted disease

There are a number of sexually transmitted diseases, including HIV/AIDS, which are not notifiable. However, various aspects of the management of HIV/AIDS are governed by statute.

- The National Health Service (Venereal Diseases) Regulations 1974 place a duty on health authorities to ensure that information on individuals suffering from sexually transmitted diseases should not be disclosed. This clearly helps to maintain the confidentiality of sufferers.
- The AIDS (Control) Act 1987 (as amended) requires health authorities to provide reports on AIDS to the Secretary of State.
- The Public Health (Infectious Diseases) Regulations 1988 (SI 1988/1546) enable local authorities to apply to a Justice of the Peace for an order to have an AIDS sufferer detained in hospital on the grounds that on leaving hospital the proper precautions to prevent the spread of infection would not be taken by the patient. There are also regulations in relation to the disposal of the body of an AIDS sufferer.

The Caldicott Report

In 1997 the Chief Medical Officer commissioned a review, under the chairmanship of Dame Fiona Caldicott, to examine the ways in which patient information was being used and the best ways to ensure that confidentiality is not undermined, particularly in relation to developments in information technology.

The Caldicott Report (1997) highlighted six key principles and made a number of recommendations.

Caldicott Principles

The six principles of the Report were:

- Justify the purpose(s) of the use of identifiable patient information.
- Do not use patient-identifiable information unless it is absolutely necessary.
- Use the minimum necessary patient-identifiable information.
- Access to patient-identifiable information should be on a strict need-to-know basis.
- Everyone with access to patient-identifiable information should be aware of their responsibilities.
- Understand and comply with the law.

A useful mnemonic, based on the name **Fiona Caldicott**, and devised by John Griffin of Thames Gateway, for remembering these principles is shown in Table 4.4.

Caldicott Guardians

One of the recommendations of the Committee was the appointment of guardians to safeguard the confidentiality of identifiable patient information.

Table 4.4 Caldicott Principles

Mnemonic for the Caldicott Principles
F ormal justification of purpose
I nformation transferred only when absolutely necessary
O nly the minimum required
N eed to know access controls
A ll to understand their responsibilities
C omply with and understand the law

Health Circular 199/012 clarifies the strategic, advisory and facilitative roles of the guardians. The guardian should be chosen from one of the following, in order of priority:

- an existing member of the management board;
- a senior health professional; or
- an individual with responsibility for promoting clinical governance within the organization.

Statutes relating to access to information

There are three Acts that are directly relevant to the issue of access to medical records.

The Data Protection Act 1984

This allows a 'data subject' to have knowledge of electronically stored information held by the 'data user'. The Data Protection (Subject Access Modification) (Health) Order 1987 (SI 1987/1903) allowing patients access to their medical records provides exceptions to access to information if the disclosure would cause serious physical or mental harm to the data subject or disclose the identity of another individual (Table 4.5).

Access to Medical Reports Act 1988

S.1 allows right of access to reports made for insurance or employment purposes and states:

Table 4.5 Exceptions to the access provisions of the Data Protection Act 1984

The access provisions do not apply if their application:
1. Would be likely to cause serious harm to the physical or mental health of the data subject; or
2. Would be likely to disclose to the data subject the identity of another individual (who has not consented to the disclosure of the information) either as a person to whom the information or part of it relates or as the source of the information or enable that identity to be deduced by the data subject either from the information itself or from a combination of that information and other information which the data subject has or is likely to have
The Data Protection (Subject Access Modification) (Health) Order 1987 (SI 1987/1903)

'It shall be the right of an individual to have access, in accordance with the provisions of this Act, to any medical report relating to the individual which is to be, or has been, supplied by a medical practitioner for employment purposes or insurance purposes.'

Access to Health Records Act 1990

This provides for access to manual information.

Section 3(1) allows access by:

1 The patient

2 A person authorized to apply on the patient's behalf

3 The person who has parental responsibility for a child

4 Where the person is incompetent at law to manage his or her affairs, the person lawfully appointed to manage them

5 The personal representative of a deceased person where the information is needed to substantiate a claim arising out of the death.

Section 5(1) is a disclaimer allowing the holder to withhold access if such access would be likely to cause serious mental or physical harm to the patient or any other individual.

Data Protection Act 1998

The Data Protection Act 1998 gives effect to the European Directive on Data Protection 1995. It came into force in March 2000 and applies to manual as well as computer records. Schedule 1, Part 1 of the Act sets out the principles with which organizations processing personal data must comply. These principles include the fairness and lawfulness of the processing, the accuracy of data, the purposes for which it is used, the time it may be retained and security arrangements (Table 4.6).

Under the Data Protection Act, individuals have specific rights. These rights include a right of subject access to the information and to take action to rectify, block, erase or destroy inaccurate data, a right to prevent processing of data likely to cause damage or distress and a right to compensation if the individual is harmed.

Offences under the Act include:

Table 4.6 The Data Protection Act Principles

- Data must be processed fairly and lawfully.
- Personal data shall be obtained only for one or more specific and lawful purposes.
- Personal data shall be adequate, relevant and not excessive in relation to the purpose(s) for which they are processed.
- Personal data shall be accurate and where necessary kept up to date.
- Personal data processed for any purpose(s) shall not be kept for longer than is necessary for that purpose.
- Personal data shall be processed in accordance with the rights of data subjects under the 1998 Data Protection Act.
- Appropriate technical and organizational measures shall be taken against unauthorized or unlawful processing of personal data and against accidental loss or destruction of, or damage to, personal data.
- Personal data shall not be transferred to a country outside the European Economic Area, unless that country or territory ensures an adequate level of protection for the rights and freedoms of data subjects in relation to the processing of personal data.

Taken from Schedule 1 Part 1 of the Data Protection Act 1998

- Unlawful obtaining and disclosure of information
- Unlawful selling of data
- Processing without notification
- Failure to notify changes of circumstances
- Failure to comply with written requests for details.

Offences are punishable with a maximum fine of £5,000 in a Magistrates' Court or an unlimited fine in the Crown Court. Both organizations and individuals can be prosecuted.

Health and Social Care Act 2001

It has been estimated that there are over 250 disease registers, probably at least 5 public health initiatives and perhaps even hundreds of research projects where access to personal data might breach confidentiality. A particular difficulty arises with the transfer of identifiable patient data to cancer registers. Such transfers may be important in managed care pathways for cancer. Patient databases are also useful for purposes of research and for disease management and planning. The Data Protection Act allows use of data for the benefit of public health without patient consent under Schedule 3. However, doubts were raised about the use of personal data in such ways without specific consent from the patient, especially after the passage of the Human Rights Act 1998. The advice from the GMC had been that such data transfer should only occur with consent or after patient identification has been removed. Parliament therefore passed the Health and Social Care Act 2001. Under s.60(1) of this Act:

'The Secretary of State may by regulations make such provision for and in connection with requiring or regulating the processing of prescribed patient information for medical purposes as he considers necessary or expedient:
(a) in the interests of improving patient care, or
(b) in the public interest.'

In May 2002 the GMC issued a statement in support of s.60 'as a temporary measure to allow essential identifiable information to be shared without consent, in tightly controlled circumstances'.

Acceptable purposes for the use of identifiable patient information as defined by the Health and Social Care Act 2001 include:
- Preventive medicine
- Medical diagnosis and research
- The provision of care and treatment
- Management of health and social care services
- Informing individuals about their physical or mental health, diagnosis of their condition or their care.

Hence, where there has been approval by Parliament or the Secretary of State under the powers created by s.60, there are no legal barriers to the transfer of patient information to organizations for the purposes specified above. A register will be maintained of all activities approved under s.60, which will be web-based and available to the public (Section 60 Register). Regulations will permit, but not require, patient information to be disclosed. Objections raised by patients should still be respected.

The Health and Social Care Act also has a provision allowing the Secretary of State, on the advice of the Patient Information Advisory Group, to introduce a legal requirement to disclose in certain circumstances. This capability exists, in rare circumstances, so as to address any currently unforeseen developments. Hence, the Health and Social Care Act 2001 may set aside the legal duty of confidentiality where the recipient satisfies the requirements specified in s.60 of the Act.

Conclusion

Doctors owe an ethical and legal responsibility to maintain patient confidentiality. Disclosure of information without the patient's consent may be justified in order to prevent harm to others or serious crime. Patients now have extensive rights to have access to, and even correct, personal data held

in manual or computer records. The handling of personal data held on disease databases and registers is now regulated by statute law.

Key points

- Patients have an ethical and legal right to confidentiality.
- Patients have extensive legal rights regarding any manual or computer records that contain personalized data, including a right to compensation where disclosure causes harm.
- There are certain statutory requirements to disclose personal information, e.g. notification of an abortion or of a serious communicable disease.
- Patient information may be disclosed to prevent crime or serious harm to others, and at the direction of a court.
- When producing medical records either manually or electronically it is important to remember that they may be read by the patient at some later date.

Clinical negligence

The aim of this chapter is to provide an understanding of when a doctor owes a duty of care to patients regarding both diagnosis and treatment, to explain how that duty of care can be breached by clinical negligence and how it is assessed by the courts.

Introduction

The law regarding negligence is developing rapidly. There are even ideas to reduce the amount of clinical litigation through 'no fault' compensation schemes. Why should the victim of negligence have to prove causation and harm? The Chief Medi-

cal Officer (CMO) issued a report, *Making Amends*, on clinical negligence reform in June 2003. In this the CMO made proposals for reform 'to ensure that the emphasis of the NHS is directed at preventing harm, reducing risks and enhancing safety so that the level of medical error is reduced. In addition there should be a "duty of candour" with immunity from disciplinary action for those reporting adverse events or medical errors (except where there is a criminal offence or where it would not be safe for the professional to continue to treat patients).'

The CMO's Report makes interesting reading for those who are involved in handling medical errors or have experienced at first hand the effects of such errors on doctors, their families, patients and relatives. Not all medical mistakes are due to medical error. Many either are caused by failures within the organization or are healthcare 'systems' failures. 'Systems failures' include e.g. access to laboratory and radiological services 'out of hours', poor medical records systems or lack of computer resources to enable rapid and comprehensive access to the results of investigations. According to the 'systems approach' medical errors often arise as a result of a number of failures within the system.

The Swiss cheese model was suggested by Professor James Reason to illustrate that for the effects of medical error to result in harm, a number of barriers and safeguards are bypassed that would normally prevent the consequences of the medical error (Fig 5.1).

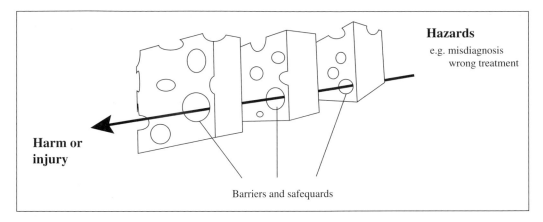

Figure 5.1. Swiss Cheese model of medical adverse events. Modified from J Reason, *BMJ* 2000;320:768–70.

Nevertheless, despite the obvious attractiveness of 'systems based' approaches to medical mishaps, it would seem that, for the foreseeable future, the management of adverse events will focus very much on 'person failure' rather than on 'systems failure'. This chapter is therefore focused on clinical negligence as it now stands. No-fault compensation, legal immunity for exercising a 'duty of candour' and a rigorous 'systems'-based approach to avoiding or reducing medical errors through risk management seems some way off.

The extent of the problem

Clinical negligence claims are a considerable financial burden on the NHS budget (Table 5.1).

Some helpful descriptions:
- Malpractice involves a breach of an ethical or professional duty, whether or not it leads to harm.
- Negligence is malpractice that results in injury to a patient.
- Rashness involves an act that a reasonable person ought not perform, or alternatively, a failure to act where the reasonable person would have acted, such that harm ensues.
- Recklessness goes beyond mere rashness, and involves negligent behaviour without due regard for the consequences, e.g. operating whilst drunk.
- Misjudgement involves an error in clinical judgement regarding either diagnosis or treatment, but does not necessarily involve negligence. However, there can be a very thin line between

Table 5.1 Clinical Negligence—facts and figures

- In 2001 the National Health Service was facing a projected clinical negligence bill of nearly £4bn.
- The actual expenditure from negligence claims was estimated at £446m in 2001/02.
- The estimated bill for actual and anticipated claims has risen sevenfold in 5 years.
- 10,000 new claims were made in 1999–2000.
- Only around 24% of claims funded by the Legal Services Commission were successful.
- Cerebral palsy and brain damage accounted for 80% of outstanding claims by value.
- For large claims (over £100,000) the average time to settlement was five and a half years.
- In 65% of settlements under £50,000, the legal and other costs actually exceeded the damages awarded.

National Audit Office 2001

misjudgement and malpractice. Lord Denning pointed out that medical treatment involves some inherent risk, and that not every error of judgement should be regarded as negligent.

Lord Denning said:

'Every surgical operation involves risks. It would be wrong, and indeed bad law, to say that simply because a misadventure or mishap occurred, the hospital and the doctors are thereby liable ... You must not, therefore, find him negligent simply because something happens to go wrong; if, for instance, one of the risks inherent in an operation actually takes place or some complication ensues which lessens or takes away the benefits that were hoped for, or if in a matter of opinion he makes an error of judgement. You should only find him guilty of negligence when he falls short of the standard of a reasonably skilful medical man, in short, when he is deserving of censure.'

Lord Denning in *Hatcher v. Black* (1954)

Recklessness can be of such a degree as to give rise to a criminal charge, e.g. for assault or murder. Negligence is usually insufficient to give rise to a criminal charge. Criminal negligence has been invoked in some homicide cases to reduce a charge of murder to one of manslaughter.

'In order to establish criminal liability, the facts must be such, that in the opinion of the jury, the negligence of the accused went beyond a mere matter of compensation between subjects and showed such disregard for the life and safety of others as to amount to a crime against the State and conduct deserving of punishment.'

Lord Chief Justice Hewart in *R v Bateman* (1925)

Mens rea and actus reus

For a doctor to be guilty of a crime it would be necessary to prove both

- *mens rea* (or a guilty mind); and
- *actus reus* (or a guilty act).

The standard of proof in criminal proceedings is proof 'beyond reasonable doubt', whereas for civil convictions it is proof 'on the balance of probabilities, i.e. where the event is more likely than not or at least 51% probable. Sometimes the courts demand a higher standard of proof in certain types of civil cases, on the basis of the principle that the more serious the wrong the higher is the standard of proof required to prove it. In 'committal' proceedings, where a person is likely to be committed to prison by a civil court (e.g. for a contempt of court), the standard of proof is as high as the criminal standard. That is because the liberty of the subject is involved—i.e. the defendant may be deprived of his liberty and sent to prison, even though the case is not a criminal one. Committal proceedings are sometimes called 'quasi-criminal'

for this reason. A person could be committed to prison for deliberately failing to obey an order of the court, because that is a type of contempt of court.

A doctor's duty of care

The Neighbour Principle

Before 1932, the duty of care in negligence was not widely defined. Matters changed after the curious case of *Donoghue v. Stevenson*. Mrs Donoghue went to a café with a friend, who bought her a bottle of ginger beer, which she consumed. She discovered a decomposed snail in the drink, and became ill. Mrs Donoghue had no direct contract with the manufacturer, so she sued in delict (the Scottish equivalent of tort in English law).

The House of Lords decided that the manufacturers had a duty of care to the consumer of their product, and awarded damages to Mrs Donoghue. This case established non-contractual liability on a sound footing. Lord Atkin laid down the principle that:

'You must take care to avoid acts or omissions which you can reasonably foresee would be likely to injure your neighbour. Who, then, in law, is my neighbour? The answer seems to be persons who are so closely and directly affected by my act that I ought reasonably to have them in contemplation as being so affected when I am directing my mind to the acts or omissions which are called in question.'

Lord Atkin in *Donoghue v Stevenson* (1932)

The two-stage test of negligence

The above test has since been regarded as too wide. Lord Wilberforce established the two-stage test of negligence.

'First, one has to ask whether, as between the alleged wrongdoer and the person who has suffered damage there is a sufficient relationship of proximity or neighbourhood such that, in the reasonable contemplation of the former, carelessness on his part may be likely to cause damage to the latter—in which case a *prima facie* duty of care arises. Secondly, if the first question is answered affirmatively, it is necessary to consider whether there are any considerations which ought to negate, or to reduce or limit the scope of the duty or the class of person to whom it is owed or the damages to which a breach of it may give rise.'

Lord Wilberforce in Anns v London Borough of Merton (1977)

The three-stage test

More recently, an additional test was applied by Lord Bridge that it should be 'just and reasonable' for the law to impose a duty of care. Hence, a claim for negligence arising from a breach of a duty of care may arise if:

(1) There is a proximate relationship between plaintiff and defendant;
(2) There is forseeability of harm to the plaintiff, to whom a duty is owed; and
(3) It is just and reasonable that a duty of care is owed in the circumstances.

Lord Bridge in Caparo Industries Plc v. Dickman (1990)

Where there may not be a duty of care: public policy considerations

The role of policy ('public policy considerations') has been recognized and may restrict, or remove, a duty of care in some circumstances (Table 5.2):

1 Where the claimant is the author of his own misfortune. This is also recognized in the common law principle of *volenti non fit injuria* (there is no actionable harm if the victim voluntarily placed himself in the way of that harm). Public policy seeks to widen that principle.
2 Where a duty of care would lead to unduly defensive practices by public bodies in the exercise of their duties. For example the mother of the last victim of the Yorkshire Ripper, Susan Hill, sued the police for negligence. The House of Lords decided that the police had no duty of care to Susan Hill,

Table 5.2 Public policy considerations and a doctor's duty of care

Exceptions to the duty of care may arise if it would:
• Lead to unduly defensive practices.
• Limit the resources available to an authority to fulfil its duties.
• Cut across a complex statutory framework set up by Parliament.
Or where:
• The claimant is responsible for his own misfortune.
• There is an alternative remedy for the claimant.

Table 5.3 Duty of care and public authorities

In the case of *X (minors) v. Bedfordshire County Council* (1995) two children brought actions for the authorities' alleged negligence in the treatment of claims of child abuse. One child was left with its parents and suffered abuse; in the other case, the child was unnecessarily taken from the parents.
The House of Lords decided that where there was a statutory discretion conferred on a public authority, nothing the authority did within the ambit of that discretion was actionable. Hence, there was no duty of care for local authorities, or the professionals they engaged, when fulfilling their public law duty towards children in need. However, the European Court went on to state that any blanket immunity for local authorities in the exercise of their statutory functions would be a violation of the right to an effective remedy under Art.13 of the Convention, and that this and other cases would need to be argued on their merits.
X (Minors) v. Bedfordshire County Council (1995) See also *Z v United Kingdom* (2001)

who was at no greater risk than any other member of the public.
3 Where an award of damages and costs against a public authority would have an adverse effect on the resources available to the authority to perform its duties (Table 5.3).
4 Where a duty of care would cut across a complex statutory framework set up by Parliament in particular circumstances, as in the case of child protection by public authorities.
5 Where there is an alternative remedy for the claimant, e.g. where there is a statutory right of

appeal or another source of compensation, e.g. the criminal injuries compensation scheme.

The 'custom test' and deviation from normal practice

The 'custom test' is one that is applied in other areas of negligence and is endorsed by Lord Clyde's dictum in the Scottish case of *Hunter v Hanley*, in which a doctor was accused of breaking a hypodermic needle whilst giving an injection.

> 'To establish liability by a doctor where deviation from normal practice is alleged, three facts require to be established. First of all it must be proved that there is a usual and normal practice; secondly it must be proved that the defender has not adopted that practice; and thirdly (and this is of crucial importance) it must be established that the course the doctor adopted is one which no professional man of ordinary skill would have taken if he had been acting with ordinary care.'
> Lord Clyde in *Hunter v Hanley* (1955)

Finally, the extent of a duty of care in negligence is a question for the court. In the case of *Hedley Byrne v Heller* (1964), the claimants sought damages for a negligent credit reference by the bank. Lord Pears stated:

> 'How wide the sphere of the duty of care in negligence is to be laid depends ultimately on the courts' assessment of the demands of society for protection from the carelessness of others.'
> Lord Pears in *Hedley Byrne v Heller* (1964)

Vicarious liability of employers

Vicarious liability is where one person is liable for the negligent acts of another. Hence, a parent may be liable for the actions of a child and an employer, e.g. an NHS Trust, for those of its employees (Table 5.4).

Two conditions must however be satisfied for employers' liability.
1 There must be an employer–employee relationship. Those working under a 'contract of service' are employees, while those under a 'contract for

Table 5.4 Long hours—a case for litigation?

An obstetric SHO was employed to work a basic 40-hour week with an additional 48 hours resident 'on-call'. He was required to work 32 hours over one particular weekend, during which he only had 30 minutes sleep. On another weekend he worked continuously for 49 hours, taking over 60 calls, and slept for only seven hours. Dr Johnstone took the Health Authority to court and successfully argued that he had suffered personal injury due to his work schedule. The Court of Appeal held that the doctor could not lawfully be required to work so much overtime, which constituted a threat to his health, and stated that it was 'a matter of grave public concern that junior doctors should be required to work such long hours without proper rest so that not only their own health may be put at risk but that of their patients as well'.
Johnstone v Bloomsbury HA (1991)

services' are independent contractors. An additional test is the degree of control exercised by the employer over the way the work is to be done.
2 The tort must be committed when the employees are acting in the course of their employment.

NHS Indemnity

NHS bodies such as NHS hospitals are vicariously liable for the negligent acts and omissions of employees. NHS Indemnity applies to the negligent acts of healthcare professionals:
• Working under a contract of employment to provide services.
• Not working under contract of employment but nevertheless contracted to provide services to persons to whom the NHS owes a duty of care.
• Where neither of the above applies but there is still a duty of care to the persons injured.
NHS Indemnity also applies to others who need not have a contract of employment and may not even be healthcare professionals, yet who owe a duty of care to the patients. These include students, medical academics with honorary contracts, voluntary workers, persons undergoing further professional education, training or examinations, students and staff working on income-generation

projects and those conducting clinical trials (with the agreement of the NHS Trust).

NHS hospital doctors are employed by the Trust to provide services and are generally covered by NHS Indemnity.

NHS Indemnity does not apply to individuals accused of criminal charges or subject to disciplinary procedures by their employer or professional body.

Also, NHS Indemnity does not cover:

- Family health-service practitioners such as GPs, general dental practitioners, pharmacists or optometrists if not directly employed by a Health Authority.
- Self-employed healthcare professionals, e.g. private psychologists.
- Employees of private hospitals.
- Local education authorities.
- Voluntary agencies.

Types of claimant in negligence cases (Table 5.5)

In addition to claims made by patients as 'primary victims', there are other potential claimants to whom a duty may be owed:

1 'Secondary victims'. A person may be a 'secondary victim' if they suffer psychiatric damage as a result of harm done to another. The conditions are that there must be:

  a Reasonable foreseeability of psychiatric illness arising from the close relationship between the claimant and the primary victim of the defendant's negligence;

  b Physical and temporal proximity between the 'secondary victim' and the accident caused by the defendant; and that

  c The psychiatric harm must arise from the claimant's sight or hearing of the event or its aftermath.

2 Employees. Employers may be responsible for psychiatric and physical injury to employees.

3 A deceased person by virtue of the Fatal Accidents Act 1976. The deceased person's personal representatives will sue on behalf of his or her estate in such a case.

4 An unborn child in respect of injuries sustained whilst in the mother's womb by virtue of the Congenital Disabilities (Civil Liability) Act 1976. This gives a right of action to a child born alive but disabled if the disability was caused during pregnancy or labour.

5 A rescuer may have a justifiable claim as the victim of negligence. A person creating a danger might be responsible for damage or injury caused to a rescuer.

Defences against liability for negligence

Limitation period

For an adult this is generally three years from the time of the alleged negligence or from the date of discovery of the harm. However, the court has discretion to extend the period. The period of limitation does not apply to children, for whom the three years start from their eighteenth birthday, or to mentally incompetent adults who are unable to manage their affairs. In cases of children severely brain-damaged since birth, there is no time-limit for bringing a claim.

Table 5.5 Potential claimants in negligence cases

- Primary victim—the patient
- Secondary victims—those suffering psychiatric harm from the incident
- Employees where the employer is responsible for psychiatric injury
- A deceased person under the Fatal Accidents Act 1976
- An unborn child under the Congenital Disabilities (Civil Liability) Act 1976
- A rescuer when the defendant was responsible for the initial danger

Table 5.6 Defences against liability for clinical negligence

- Expiry of limitation period
- Consent and agreement to undergo risk
- Contributory negligence by the claimant, e.g. failure to follow medical advice

Consent

A patient who has agreed to run the risk of harm cannot bring proceedings relating to damage caused by taking that risk. However, consent may be vitiated by undue coercion, fraud or misrepresentation. Defective consent may obviate charges of assault and battery but may still give rise to claims in civil negligence. A signed consent form is not necessarily proof that the patient has been adequately informed.

Contributory negligence

The claimant may himself contribute to the injury by, for example, ignoring medical advice. Hence, according to the Law Reform (Contributory Negligence) Act 1945 s 1(1):

'Where any person suffers damage as the result of his own fault and partly the fault of another person or persons, a claim in respect of that damage shall not be defeated by reason of the fault of the person suffering the damage but the damages recoverable in respect thereof shall be reduced to such extent as the court thinks just and equitable having regard to the claimant's share in the responsibility for the damage.'

For example, in the case of *Barrett v Ministry of Defence* (1995), a sailor became drunk and passed out. As a result of inadequate treatment he choked to death on his own vomit. His widow successfully sued the Navy for negligence. The Court of Appeal held that, while the Navy did not owe a duty to prevent his drunkenness, having found him comatose it had negligently failed to seek medical assistance. However, the sailor was two-thirds to blame for his own death, and the damages were reduced accordingly.

Determination of a claim for negligence (Table 5.7)

Establishing a duty of care

The civil liability of doctors was summarized in *R v. Batemen (1925)*.

Table 5.7 Determination of a claim for negligence

In order to substantiate a claim for negligence it is necessary to establish:
(a) A duty of care
(b) A breach of that duty
(c) A causal relationship between the breach of duty and harm caused to the plaintiff
(d) Proximity and foreseeability of harm
(e) Loss and damage arising from the injury
(f) That it is just and reasonable for a duty of care to exist in the circumstances.

'If a person holds himself out as possessing special skill and knowledge and he is consulted, as possessing such skill and knowledge, by or on behalf of the patient he owes a duty to the patient to use due caution in undertaking the treatment. If he accepts the responsibility and undertakes the treatment and the patient submits to his direction and treatment accordingly, he owes a duty to the patient to use diligence, care, knowledge, skill and caution in administering the treatment. No contractual relation is necessary, nor is it necessary that the service is rendered for reward.'

A duty of care to patients is transferred upon a doctor taking up an NHS appointment. General practitioners assume responsibility for patients when they accept them on to their lists. They may opt for the provision of additional services such as maternity services. A doctor in private practice may also have entered into a contractual arrangement with the patient, though the professional obligation of the doctor is independent of any contract or monetary transaction. For the same reason, doctors performing 'Good Samaritan' acts in emergencies are also expected to provide acceptable standards of medical care, having due regard to the circumstances.

Demonstrating a breach of duty

Individual doctors may be responsible for health care; but patients are often managed within a multidisciplinary setting. Actions taken against indi-

Table 5.8 The *Bolam* case

Mr Bolam was a manic depressive who underwent electro-convulsive therapy. He was not given muscle relaxants and sustained severe fractures during the ensuing seizures caused by the ECT. He had not been apprised of the risks or of the possibility of the use of drugs and other restraining measures to minimize the possibility of fracture. However, at that time the use of such measures was not routine or generally accepted practice.

Bolam v. Friern Hospital Management Committee (1957)

Table 5.9 The *Bolam* Principle

'The test is the standard of the ordinary skilled man exercising and professing to have that special skill. A man need not possess the highest expert skill; it is well-established that it is sufficient if he exercises the ordinary skill of an ordinary competent man exercising that particular art.

[A doctor] is not guilty of negligence if he has acted in accordance with a practice accepted as proper by a reasonable body of medical men skilled in that particular art . . . Putting it the other way round, a man is not negligent, if he is acting in accordance with such a practice, merely because there is a body of opinion who would take a contrary view.'

Mr Justice McNair in *Bolam v. Friern Hospital Management Committee* (1957)

vidual doctors alone are less likely to succeed than claims made against NHS Trusts.

Bolam Principle

In most cases of clinical negligence it is usually a straightforward matter to establish that the doctor owed a duty of care. The difficulty is mainly to prove that the standard of care owed was breached. The current principal test of negligence was established as a result of the *Bolam* case (Table 5.8).

According to the time-honoured *Bolam Principle* a doctor is not guilty of negligence if he has acted in accordance with a practice accepted as proper by a responsible body of medical men skilled in that particular art; he is not negligent if he is acting in accordance with such a practice, merely because there is a body of opinion that takes the contrary view (Table 5.9).

Lord Scarman in *Maynard v. West Midlands RHA* (1984) stated that a doctor who professes to exercise a special skill must demonstrate the ordinary skill of that speciality. The case involved a failure in the diagnosis of tuberculosis. Furthermore a judge's 'preference' for one body of distinguished medical opinion over another equally distinguished body of opinion was not sufficient to establish negligence (Table 5.10).

Lord Edmund-Davies in *Whitehouse v Jordan* (1981) upheld the *Bolam* Principle but pointed out that clinical judgement may be negligent if it gives rise to an error that would not have been made by a reasonably competent practitioner professing

Table 5.10 The *Maynard* test

'In the realm of diagnosis and treatment negligence is not established by preferring one respectable body of professional opinion to another. Failure to exercise the ordinary skill of a doctor (in the appropriate speciality, if he be a specialist) is necessary.'

Lord Scarman in *Maynard v West Midlands Regional Health Authority* (1984)

skill in the same speciality and acting with ordinary care. The case involved the use of obstetrical forceps, and Lord Edmund-Davies stated:

'. . . other acts or omissions in the case of exercising "clinical judgment" may be so glaringly below proper standards as to make a finding of negligence inevitable'.

However, *Bolam* has been modified to some extent by the case of *Bolitho*, where it was decided that the court is not bound to hold that the doctor escapes liability for diagnosis or treatment simply because there are medical experts who agree that the defendant's conduct was in accord with sound medical practice (Table 5.11).

The court must be satisfied that the medical opinion has a logical basis.

'In particular, in cases involving, as they often do, the weighing of risks and benefits, the judge,

Table 5.11 The *Bolitho* case

A two-year-old boy, Patrick Bolitho, with a previous history of croup was admitted to hospital under Drs H and R. He suffered two short episodes of dyspnoea. Dr H was called in the first instance and delegated to Dr R in the second instance. On the second occasion neither doctor saw the patient. The patient then had a cardio-respiratory arrest resulting in severe brain damage and died.

The case revolved around whether an intubation after the second bout of dyspnoea would have prevented the eventual cardio-respiratory arrest. It was decided that even if Dr H had attended on the second occasion, she would not have intubated the patient, and that this failure to act would not have been negligent. While intubation might well have prevented the final calamity, it was not without risk. The decision was upheld by the House of Lords.

Bolitho v Hackney Health Authority (1997)

before accepting a body of opinion as being responsible, reasonable or respectable, will need to be satisfied that, in forming their views, the experts have directed their minds to the question of comparative risks and benefits and have reached a defensible view in the matter.'

Lord Browne-Wilkinson in *Bolitho v Hackney Health Authority* (1997)

However, it will rarely be correct for a judge to regard as unreasonable the genuinely held views of a competent medical expert and it will rarely be the case that the professional opinion is 'not capable of withstanding logical analysis'. The balancing of risks and benefits is a matter of clinical judgement, a judgement that a court would not normally make. It is only when an opinion cannot be logically supported that it will cease to be the benchmark for assessing the defendant's conduct.

The *Bolam* test does not necessarily require a large body of opinion. The case of *De Frietas v O'Brien* (1995) gives some comfort to the super-specialist who may be called upon to undertake high-risk cases. In this case, a spinal surgeon—one of only about 11 in the country—maintained that the surgery he performed was in line with what his fellow

surgeons would consider clinically justifiable, whereas the plaintiffs claimed that ordinary orthopaedic surgeons would not have operated. The Court of Appeal held that the *Bolam* test did not require the body of responsible opinion to be large.

Causation

For a claim of negligence to succeed, it is necessary to show that the acts or omissions of the doctor(s) led to harm that the patient would not have suffered 'but for' the negligent behaviour. Hence the claimant must establish that 'but for' the negligence he would not have suffered the injury or a particular aggravation of the injury. This is often referred to by lawyers as the 'but for' test of causality.

In rare instances causation can be shown on the basis of the legal principle called *res ipsa loquitur* ('the thing speaks for itself'). An example is found in the case of *Cassidy v Ministry of Health* (1951), where the plaintiff underwent an operation on two of his fingers for Dupuytren's contracture, but ended up with a useless hand. The plaintiff was successful simply on the basis that

'That should not have happened if due care had been used. Explain it if you can.'

Causation is not established if the injury would have occurred in any event. For example, a man presented to hospital with stomach pains and vomiting. The duty doctor refused to examine him and sent him home. He died of arsenic poisoning five hours later. The hospital was unsuccessfully sued. The medical evidence was that he would probably have died even with prompt treatment (Table 5.12).

Causation may be difficult to establish even in the face of malpractice if either there were other possible causes of the injury or another intervening event or events that broke the chain of causality between the doctor's action and the injury—what is sometimes termed a *novus actus interveniens* ('a new intervening act').

An example of the difficulty in proving causality is seen in the case of *Wilsher v Essex Health Authority* (1988).

Table 5.12 Failure to diagnose arsenic poisoning

Three nightwatchmen drank some tea around 5 a.m. and subsequently started to vomit. They later walked into Casualty around 8 a.m. One man appeared ill, and lay down. Another man told the nurse that they had vomited after drinking tea. She telephoned the Casualty officer, who was himself unwell. He said they should go home and call their own doctors, but did not see the men. The deceased died several hours later of arsenic poisoning.

Barnett v Chelsea and Kensington Hospital Management Committee (1969)

Table 5.13 A case of retrolental fibroplasia—but causation through negligence could not be proved

Baby Wilsher was born in 1978, almost three months prematurely, as a 'very floppy blue baby'. He was admitted to the Special Care Baby Unit on oxygen delivered by a facemask. A junior doctor mistakenly placed a catheter into the umbilical vein for arterial blood gas analysis. This error was overlooked by both a senior registrar and a consultant radiologist. Both the resident and the senior registrar had been working excessive hours, having been 'on call' every second night and weekend. The catheter was replaced after 24 hours by the senior registrar, but was again inserted into the umbilical vein rather than the artery. Baby Wilsher therefore received excessive oxygen for approximately 32 hours, and developed retrolental fibroplasia (RLF) and near-total blindness. The Court of Appeal held that:
'a health authority which so conducts its hospital that it fails to provide doctors of sufficient skill and experience to give the treatment offered at the hospital may be directly liable in negligence to the patient . . . I can see no reason why, in principle, the health authority should not be so liable if its organization is at fault.'

Wilsher v Essex Health Authority (1986)

This case is also important in relation to the liability of inexperienced doctors (see Table 5.13).

In the case of *Wilsher v Essex Health Authority*, although the placement of the catheter was held to be negligent, it could not be proved that excess oxygen caused the blindness.

'There was no satisfactory evidence that excess oxygen is more likely than any of four candidates to have caused RLF in this baby.'

The eggshell skull rule

If some harm was foreseeable, the defendant is liable for the full extent of the claimant's injuries even if the victim is unusually susceptible to injury.

Lord Justice Mackinnon held that:

'One who is guilty of negligence to another must put up with idiosyncrasies of his victim that increase the likelihood or extent of damage to him; it is no answer to a claim for a fractured skull that its owner had an unusually fragile one.'

Lord Justice Mackinnon in *Owens v. Liverpool Corporation* (1938)

Proximity and foreseeability of harm

The harm must have been reasonably close and foreseeable in relation to the act or omission. Where the omission is a failure to make a diagnosis, the assumption is that the patient would have been properly treated by a reasonably skilled practitioner, had the correct diagnosis been made.

In *Penny and Others v East Kent Health Authority* (2000), several women had undergone false negative cervical smear tests but subsequently went on to develop cancer. The Court held that a reasonably competent cytoscreener should have recognized Mrs Penny's smear as being abnormal and ought to have passed it on for further assessment by a cytopathologist. Had the smear been regarded as abnormal, Mrs Penny would have had further follow-up, the carcinoma would have been discovered sooner, and she would have received earlier treatment (which would presumably have been successful).

It is the foreseeability of harm, and not necessarily knowledge of a particular injury that is required. In *Margereson v Roberts* (1996), the defendant had played as a child in the 1930s in the grounds of an asbestos factory and subsequently developed the fatal lung condition, mesothelioma.

Mesothelioma was unforeseeable prior to research published on this condition in 1960. However, the Court of Appeal held that it had been known since the turn of the century that breathing asbestos dust created a risk of physical harm, and that was sufficient.

Furthermore, where negligence has occurred, a wrongdoer ought to foresee that the victim may require medical treatment, and he may be liable for the consequences of that treatment. In the case of *Robinson v Post Office* (1974), a man slipped on a ladder at work because of oil on a step, suffering a minor injury. He went to hospital and was given an anti-tetanus injection, to which he reacted and developed encephalitis. According to Lord Justice Orr, the employers were responsible for both the minor injury and the subsequent encephalitis.

Novus actus interveniens

In establishing causation the Court must decide if any other intervening act (*novus actus interveniens*) breaks the chain of causation, or whether the ultimate damage was a direct and foreseeable consequence of the original negligence. The intervening act may be an act of nature, of a third party or the claimant himself (Table 5.14).

Public policy: Is it just and reasonable to impose a duty of care?

There are situations in which the courts are reluctant to impose a duty of care. This usually applies to public bodies, where to do so might lead to an increase in litigation and impair the due exercise of the defendant's proper role. For example, it was held that the police did not have a duty of care to individual members of the public to prevent murder in the case of the Yorkshire Ripper who killed a number of women over several years (see *Hill v Chief Constable of West Yorkshire* (1989)).

Judge Edwards held that the coastguard did not owe a duty of care to mariners in *Skinner v Secretary for Transport* (1995). It would be against the public interest for resources to be diverted from sea rescues to the defending of possible claims.

Table 5.14 Chains of causality

A neurotic man sustained head injuries in the course of his work for which his employers were liable. He became increasingly anxious and depressed, and committed suicide eighteen months later. His wife sued under the Fatal Accidents Act 1976 and won. Her loss was a foreseeable result of the accident, and the 'eggshell rule' applied, even though suicide was then a crime.

Pigney v Pointers Transport (1957)

A woman injured her neck and had to wear a cervical collar. This interfered with her ability to wear glasses, and she subsequently fell down some steps. It was held that there was liability both for the original and the subsequent injuries, since the original injury could foreseeably affect a person's ability to deal with the vicissitudes of life and cause another injury.

Wieland v Cyril Lord Carpets (1969)

A man negligently set fire to his house with a blowlamp. A fireman was injured while fighting the fire, and sued for his injuries. The House of Lords held that he should succeed, as his injuries were a foreseeable result of the man's negligence, and it was not relevant that he was a fireman expected to take risks in the line of duty.

Ogwo v Taylor (1987)

Conversely, the ambulance service was held liable for failure to reach a woman suffering from an acute asthmatic attack in time, despite telling the doctor that they were 'on their way'. As a result of the delay she suffered serious mental and physical harm, and successfully sued the ambulance service. The Court of Appeal held in *Kent v Griffiths* (2000) that the acceptance of the call established a duty of care, and it was neither unjust nor unreasonable to impose such a duty. If the wrong information had not been given that the ambulance was on its way, the doctor or family could have made other arrangements for transfer to hospital.

Negligence and inexperienced doctors

An inexperienced or junior doctor is judged by the same standards as the doctor of ordinary skill, even though the degree of skill is generally lower for a novice compared to an experienced clinician.

In the case of *Wilsher v Essex Health Authority* (Table 5.13), the Court held that the doctor's duty of care was assessed in relation to the post held, not the particular experience of the doctor within that post. Junior doctors are expected to seek help when necessary, and to be adequately supervised by more senior colleagues.

In the case of *Jones v Manchester Corporation* (1952), an inexperienced junior doctor wrongly administered an anaesthetic, causing the patient to die. It was held by Lord Denning that:

'It would be in the highest degree unjust that hospital authorities, by getting inexperienced doctors to perform their duties for them, without adequate supervision, should be able to throw all the responsibility on to those doctors as if they were fully experienced practitioners.'

Consent and negligence

A doctor may legally provide treatment with the patient's consent. Without such consent a doctor risks criminal prosecution for assault, or even accusations of battery (battery requires some kind of touching, whereas assault can occur even if the victim is not touched). Consent requires that the patient is informed in broad terms of the proposed treatment. Failure adequately to warn of the risks and benefits of and alternatives to therapy may be held negligent, as in the case of *Chatterton v. Gerson* (Table 5.15).

Assault and battery are forms of trespass to the person and actionable *per se* without proof of loss or damage. An action in negligence, however, requires proof of loss or damage. Assault and battery are also criminal offences. The decision in *Chatterton* was therefore of some importance to healthcare professionals.

However, consent may be vitiated if it is obtained through fraud or misrepresentation of the nature of the treatment.

'If there was real consent to treatment, it mattered not whether the doctor was in breach of his duty to give the patient the appropriate information before that consent was given. Real consent provides a complete defence to a claim based on

Table 5.15 Inadequate consent: negligence not trespass

The claimant was being treated for chronic pain around a previous hernia operation scar. The first attempt at treatment had only been partially successful, and the patient sought a second option. She had an injection, which failed to relieve her pain but rendered her right leg numb and caused impaired mobility. She argued that her consent was vitiated by her not being told of the risk of numbness as a side-effect.
Mr Justice Bristow said:

'In my judgement once the patient is informed in broad terms of the nature of the procedure which is intended, and gives her consent, that consent is real, and the cause of the action on which to base a claim for failure to go into the risks and implications is negligence, not trespass. Of course, if information is withheld in bad faith, the consent will be vitiated by fraud . . . in my judgement it would be very much against the interests of justice if actions which are really based on a failure by the doctor to perform his duty adequately to inform were pleaded in trespass.'
Mr Justice Bristow in *Chatterton v Gerson* (1981)

Table 5.16 The case of *Freeman v Home Office* (1984)

David Freeman was a prisoner serving a life sentence at HM Prison Wakefield. He was given various drugs under the direction of Dr Xavier (Stelazine, Modecate and Serenace). Freeman claimed that he had not consented to the administration of these drugs and had 'actively resisted it, but was overcome forcibly by the said medical officer and/or prison officers'. The Court of Appeal accepted that despite the circumstances, David Freeman had consented to receiving the medication as a matter of fact.

the tort of trespass to the person. Consent would not be real if procured by fraud or misrepresentation, but subject to this and subject to the patient having been informed in broad terms of the nature of the treatment, consent in fact amounts to consent in law.'
Sir John Donaldson MR in *Freeman v. Home Office* (1984)

Table 5.17 The *Sidaway* case (1985)

Mrs Sidaway complained of recurring pains in her neck, shoulder and arms caused by spinal nerve-root compression. She underwent spinal decompression at Bethlem Royal Hospital in 1974. The risk of root damage was put at 1–2%. The risk of spinal cord damage was considerably less. Post-operatively she suffered considerable disability and partial paralysis. Mrs Sidaway sued the hospital and the executors of the surgeon, who had died by the time the case came to court in 1984. She claimed that she had not been warned of the possibility of spinal cord damage; had she been warned, she would not have agreed to the operation. Her case was dismissed by both the High Court and the Court of Appeal. Although there was insufficient evidence that the surgeon had actually failed to warn her of the operative risks, the case eventually went to the House of Lords. The core issue was whether the neurosurgeon would have been negligent in failing adequately to inform her of the risks of cord damage.

Sidaway v Governors of the Bethlem Royal Hospital and the Maudsley Hospital (1985)

Table 5.18 Failure to warn of risks: *Rogers v Whittaker* — an Australian case

A patient underwent an operation to remove scar tissue from one eye in order to improve vision. The patient had been particularly concerned about the possibility of accidentally losing the vision in her 'good eye', though not specifically as a result of the operation. The chances of her suffering a rare complication known as sympathetic ophthalmitis, in which the 'good eye' would be damaged as a result of surgery to the other eye, was estimated as 1 in 14,000 or greater. The operation was correctly performed, but she suffered sympathetic ophthalmitis and became blind within a year. While it was not the general professional practice to tell patients of such a low risk of blindness, the doctor was found in breach of his duty, since the patient had specifically voiced concern about her fears of losing the sight of the good eye.

Rogers v Whittaker (1992)

In general a doctor is fulfilling his duty to inform the patient if he acts in accordance with a competent and responsible body of medical opinion. However, the court may determine that a piece of information was so obviously necessary for proper consent that failure to disclose would invalidate the consent and that a doctor failing to provide this information would be failing in his duty of care to the patient (Table 5.17: *Sidaway* 1985), a case seen in the chapter on consent.

However, while in UK law it is not deemed necessary to detail every possible side-effect of treatment, a doctor may be in breach of his duty of care if he fails to answer truthfully questions put to him by the patient, unless the doctor feels that in the circumstances the information would be demonstrably harmful to the patient's physical or mental health. This has been termed a doctor's 'therapeutic privilege' (see *Sidaway*).

At present what constitutes adequate information is usually determined by how a responsible body of medical opinion would advise or inform a patient. However, in Australia the criterion is what

the patient (not doctors) would regard as reasonable, as is seen in the case of *Rogers v Whitaker* (Table 5.18*)*.

Hence, in the future, the standard could shift towards what a reasonable patient would require in order to exercise their right of self-determination.

For a successful claim in negligence regarding consent it is necessary for the claimant to prove that not only was the doctor negligent in portraying the risks but also that, had the risks been known, the patient would not have undergone the treatment.

There are a number of important practical aspects of consent that can be learnt from *Sidaway* (1985):

• The extent of disclosure of risks in any particular situation is a matter of clinical judgement.

• Non disclosure will usually be decided on the basis of expert medical evidence, applying the *Bolam* Principle.

• However, there may be certain circumstances where the operation involves a substantial risk of grave harm, such that 'the judge might in certain circumstances come to the conclusion that disclosure of a particular risk was so obviously necessary to an informed choice on the part of the patient that no reasonably prudent medical man would fail to make it' (Lord Bridge).

• The patient can be expected to take an active and responsible part in discussion of the risks and benefits of a treatment.

'If a patient knows that a major operation may entail serious consequences, the patient cannot complain of lack of information unless the patient asks in vain for more information or unless there is some danger which by its nature or magnitude or for some other reasons requires to be separately taken into account by the patient in order to reach a balanced judgement in deciding whether or not to submit to the operation' (Lord Templeman).

• The advice given by the doctor ought to be directed toward the patient's best clinical interests.

'An obligation to give a patient all the information available to the doctor would often be inconsistent with the doctor's contractual obligation to have regard to the patient's best interests. Some information might confuse, other information might alarm a particular patient. Whenever the occasion arises for the doctor to tell the patient the results of the doctor's diagnosis, the possible methods of treatment and the advantages and disadvantages of the recommended treatment, the doctor must decide in the light of his training and experience and in the light of his knowledge of the patient what should be said and how it should be said' (Lord Templeman).

• The doctor ought also to provide balanced advice.

'If the doctor making a balanced judgement advises the patient to submit to the operation, the patient is entitled to reject that advice for reasons which are rational, or irrational, or for no reason. The duty of the doctor in these circumstances, subject to his overriding duty to have regard to the best interests of the patient, is to provide the patient with information which will enable the patient to make a balanced judgement, if the patient chooses to make a balanced

judgement. A patient may make an unbalanced judgement because he is deprived of adequate information. A patient may also make an unbalanced judgement if he is provided with too much information and is made aware of possibilities which he is not capable of assessing because of his lack of medical training, his prejudices or his personality' (Lord Templeman).

• A doctor has a 'therapeutic privilege'.

'[where] a reasonable medical assessment of the patient would have indicated to the doctor that disclosure would have posed a serious threat of psychological detriment to the patient' (Lord Scarman).

• It is for the court to decide whether the doctor has acted in breach of his duty.

'This result is achieved first by emphasis on the patient's "right of self-determination" and secondly by the "prudent patient" test. If the doctor omits to warn where the risk is such that in the court's view a prudent person in the patient's position would have regarded it as significant, the doctor is liable'. (Lord Scarman).

• However,

'If the doctor admits or the court finds that on the prudent patient test he should have disclosed the risk, he has available the defence that he reasonably believed it to be against the best interest of his patient to disclose it. Here also medical evidence, including the evidence of the doctor himself, will be vital' (Lord Scarman).

• When a patient of apparently sound mind asks questions about risks involved in a particular treatment, the doctor's duty must be to answer both as truthfully and as fully as the questioner requires (Lord Bridge).

Conclusion

The law in relation to consent is succinctly summarized in the case of *Chester v Afshar* (2002).

'The law is designed to require doctors properly to inform their patients of the risks attendant on their treatment and to answer questions put to them as to that treatment and its dangers, such answers to be judged in the context of good professional practice, which has tended to a greater degree of frankness over the years, with more respect being given to patient autonomy. The object is to enable the patient to decide whether or not to run the risks of having that operation at that time. If the doctor's failure to take that care results in her consenting to an operation to which she would not otherwise have given her consent, the purpose of that rule would be thwarted if he were not to be held responsible when the very risk about which he failed to warn her materializes and causes her an injury which she would not have suffered then and there.'

Keypoints

- Claims of negligence against doctors are common and rising.
- Not all negligence is due to doctors' errors—some is due to 'systems' failure.
- Negligence can arise in relation to investigation, treatment and consent.
- Consent requires information to be given to the patient, especially if the patient seeks information, and, unless it would harm the patient, failure to give the information may give rise to a claim for negligence.

Part 3

Mental Health

Chapter 6

Mental health

Learning Objectives

Core knowledge
- Overall scope and functions of mental health legislation
- Basic legal definitions of mental illness and disorder
- Sections 2 and 3 regarding compulsory detention and treatment

Clinical application
- Criteria for compulsory detention and treatment

Background principles
- Purpose of Mental Health legislation
- Millan principles
- Human rights issues regarding compulsory detention and treatment

No other aspect of health care is so affected by the law on a daily basis as mental health. Psychiatrists must have a detailed working knowledge of the Mental Health Act in relation to the compulsory detention and treatment of patients who may be a risk to themselves or to others. To deprive patients of their freedom and impose compulsory treatment raises profound ethical questions and human rights issues.

Mental health legislation is complex, and gives rise to numerous cases for Judicial Review every year. The Scottish Parliament recently passed the Scottish Mental Health Care and Treatment Act in 2003. The Westminster Parliament put forward a draft Mental Health Act in June 2002. This met with criticism in respect of its proposed detention of patients with severe personality disorders even if they had not committed a crime and of its proposed extension of compulsory treatment to those living in the community. There were also concerns about safeguarding patients' rights and the risk of increasing the public stigma attaching to mental illness and the risks psychiatric patients posed to the public.

Mental Health Act 1983 (England and Wales)

Background to mental health legislation

Most doctors will be involved in the management of acutely disturbed psychiatric patients at some time. The care of such patients will mainly involve psychiatrists, but may also include casualty officers, general practitioners and hospital doctors. Table 6.1 shows the extent of mental health problems

Mental Health legislation includes powers that may significantly restrict the liberty and activities of individuals, particularly in relation to their freedom to accept or refuse medical treatment.

There were about 20 Acts of Parliament between 1808 and 1981 dealing with mentally disordered patients. However, the first comprehensive piece of Mental Health Legislation was the 1959 Mental

Table 6.1 Mental illness statistics

Mental Health: the size of the problem

- 1 in 4 people will experience some kind of mental health problem in the course of a year.
- 1 in 6 people will have depression at some point in their life.
- Depression is most common in people aged 25–44 years.
- 1 in 10 people are likely to have a 'disabling anxiety disorder' at some stage in their life.
- 1 in 100 suffer from schizophrenia and 1 in 100 from manic depression.
- 20% of women and 14% of men in England have some form of mental illness.
- Men are three times more likely than women to have alcohol dependence and twice as likely to be dependent on drugs.
- 15% of pre-school children will have mild mental health problems and 7% will have severe mental health problems.
- 15% of people over 65 have depression.
- Up to 670,000 people in the UK have some form of dementia.
- 5% of people over 65 and 10 to 20% of people over 80 have dementia.

Suicide

- There are approximately 5,000 suicides per year in England.
- 75% of all suicides are by men.
- Suicide is the commonest cause of death in men under 35.
- 20% of all deaths in young people are by suicide.
- 17% of all suicides are by people aged 65 or over.
- Between 1971 and 1996 the suicide rate for women in the UK almost halved, while that for men almost doubled.

Self-harm

- 142,000 hospital admissions each year in England and Wales are the result of deliberate self-harm.
- Self-harm is more common in women than in men.

Mental health and crime

- 10–20% of young people involved in criminal activity are thought to have a 'psychiatric disorder'.
- In England and Wales an estimated 39% of the sentenced population have mental health problems.

The costs of mental ill health

- The total cost of mental health problems in England has been estimated at £32 billion. More than a third of this cost (almost £12 billion) is attributed to lost employment and productivity.
- Over 91 million working days are lost through mental ill health every year. Half of the days lost through mental illness are due to anxiety and stress conditions.

Sources: The Mental Health Foundation and MIND

Health Act, based upon the recommendations of the Royal Commission chaired by Lord Eustace Percy. This Act was amended and updated in the Mental Health Act 1983 ('MHA'). There are approximately 44,000 patients detained in hospital for assessment and treatment for mental disorder each year under the Act, of which about 12,000 are detained in hospital at any one time.

The MHA is seen as falling short of what is now needed for the care of the mentally ill in a modern context. The Government issued a White Paper in December 2000 entitled 'Reforming The Mental Health Act' that sets out its proposals for new legislation.

The MHA only allows compulsory treatment in hospital, whereas the majority of patients are now treated in the community. This means that community-based patients can refuse treatment that may be necessary to prevent harm to themselves or to others. Lives have sometimes been put at risk through suicide or homicide, as in the Clunis case (see Table 6.2).

In a significant departure from the MHA, the White Paper proposes to strengthen and protect the public from dangerous patients suffering from personality disorders (Table 6.3).

At present many patients with personality disorder are not detained in hospital because their condition is regarded as untreatable. The proposed definition of mental disorder will include personality disorder. Such patients could be detained under the proposed legislation if they pose a serious risk of harm to others. Nevertheless, the majority of mentally ill patients do not pose a risk either to themselves or to others, and the deprivation of their liberty is a serious step requiring special safe-

Table 6.2 The Clunis case

> Mr Jonathan Zito was fatally stabbed in the eye by a paranoid schizophrenic, Christopher Clunis, as he stood on the platform at Finsbury Park underground station in north London.
>
> Mr Clunis pleaded guilty to manslaughter on the grounds of diminished responsibility. He is now detained indefinitely at Rampton secure hospital. The Court of Appeal held that in formulating the Mental Health Act 1983 Parliament had not intended to create wide-ranging responsibilities on health authorities, professionals and others for actions carried out by patients such as Clunis, who was held to have known that his actions were wrong.
>
> This murder had a high public profile and was instrumental in prompting a review of aftercare in the community and the introduction of Supervision Registers. An inquiry into the case highlighted the failures of various health and social service departments and found that no agency had an overall view of the needs of Christopher Clunis or of the risk he posed to the public.
>
> Zito's wife Jayne Zito began a campaign to change the law so that patients who were not formally detained could nevertheless be forced to take their medicine in the community. However, the powers of supervised discharge under the Mental Health (Patients in the Community) Act 1995 fall short of this because:
> - There remains no power to give compulsory treatment under supervised discharge.
> - Supervised discharge only applies to parties discharged from s.3 of the MHA 1983 and cannot be imposed on a patient in the community.

Table 6.3 Proposals in the White Paper on reform of the Mental Health Act 1983

> The Government White Paper proposes new mental health legislation. It is not yet law, but may well reflect future legislation in relation to the reform of the Mental Health Act 1983.
>
> The main proposals set out in the White paper relate to:
> - A new definition of mental disorder
> - New powers for compulsory treatment in the community
> - Wider powers of detention
> - Statutory requirements to develop and review care plans
> - A new tribunal to determine all long-term use of compulsory powers
> - A new right to independent advocacy
> - New safeguards for patients with long-term incapacity.

guards that the Government intends to improve through legislation.

Introduction to the Mental Health Act 1983

The MHA is a complex piece of legislation, and is divided into 10 parts:

Part I (s.1)	Scope of the Act (provides basic definitions)
Part II (ss.2 to 34)	Compulsory admission to hospital and guardianship
Part III (ss.35 to 55)	Patients remanded to hospital in relation to criminal proceedings
Part IV (ss.56 to 64)	Statutory provisions about consent to treatment
Part V (ss.65 to 79)	Role and function of mental health review tribunals
Part VI (ss.80 to 92)	Transfers of patients and the return of patients who are absent without leave
Part VII (ss.93 to 113)	Management of the property and affairs of patients
Part VIII (ss.114 to 115)	Miscellaneous functions of local authorities and the Secretary of State
Part IX (ss.126 to 130)	Criminal offences, such as forgery, ill treatment of patients and false documentation
Part X (ss.131 to 149)	Miscellaneous matters, including censoring correspondence and dealing with patients found in public places. It also gives statutory protection from litigation for acts done in pursuance of the Act.

Table 6.4 Mental Health Act 1983: Summary of sections

Section 1.	Scope of the Act and basic definitions
Section 2.	Admission for assessment
Section 3.	Admission for treatment
Section 4.	Emergency admission for assessment
Section 5.	Holding a person already admitted voluntarily
Section 7.	Guardianship
Section 17.	Authorized leave
Section 35.	Remand by a court for reports
Section 36.	Remand by a court for treatment
Section 56.	Scope of consent to treatment provisions
Section 57.	Treatment requiring consent and a second opinion
Section 58.	Treatment requiring consent or a second opinion
Section 63.	Treatment for mental disorder not covered by s.57 and s.58
Section 72.	Mental Health Review Tribunal's powers and duties to discharge
Section 117.	Aftercare arrangements
Section 135.	Warrant to enter premises and remove a patient
Section 136.	Removing a mentally ill person from a public place to a place of safety

A summary of the important sections of the Act for medical practitioners is shown in Table 6.4.

Scope of the Act and definitions (Part I)

The MHA concerns the admission to hospital, assessment and treatment of those with mental disorder and the management of their property.

Mental disorder

Mental disorder is defined as:

'Mental illness, arrested or incomplete development of mind, psychopathic disorder and any other disorder or disability of mind'.

The term 'mental illness' is not specifically defined in the Act but has its usual clinical meaning (Table 6.5).

The White Paper proposes a much broader definition of mental disorder to cover 'any disability or

Table 6.5 Meaning of 'mental disorder' in the Mental Health Act 1983

Mental disorder means 'mental illness, arrested or incomplete development of mind, psychopathic disorder and any other disorder or disability of mind'. Mental disorder is subdivided into 5 categories:
- **Mental illness**
A significant omission in the MHA is that there is no specific definition of mental illness as such.
- **Mental impairment**
Means 'a state of arrested or incomplete development of mind (not amounting to severe mental impairment) which includes significant impairment of intelligence and social functioning and is associated with abnormally aggressive or seriously irresponsible conduct on the part of the person concerned'.
- **Severe mental impairment**
Defined as 'a state of arrested or incomplete development of mind which includes severe impairment of intelligence and social functioning and is associated with abnormally aggressive or seriously irresponsible conduct on the part of the person concerned'.
- **Psychopathic disorder**
Means 'a persistent disorder or disability of mind (whether or not including significant impairment of intelligence) which results in abnormally aggressive or seriously irresponsible conduct on the part of the person concerned'.
- **'Any other disorder or disability of mind'**
This is a non-specific catch-all phrase.
The MHA is clear that a person must not be deemed to have mental disorder 'by reason only of promiscuity or other immoral conduct, sexual deviancy or dependence on alcohol or drugs'.

disorder of mind or brain, whether permanent or temporary, which results in an impairment or disturbance of mental functioning'.

Compulsory admission and guardianship procedures (Part II)

Admission for assessment (Section 2)

S.2 authorizes the compulsory detention of a patient for assessment on the recommendation of two medical practitioners, one of whom must be approved under s.12 of the Act and is usually a consultant psychiatrist. The other doctor should have previous acquaintance with the patient, and will often be a general practitioner.

The criteria for the detention of a patient are:

a That he is suffering from a mental disorder of a nature or degree that warrants the detention of the patient in a hospital for assessment (or for assessment followed by treatment) for at least a limited period; and

b That he ought to be so detained in the interests of his own health or safety or with a view to the protection of others.

Sexual deviancy and abuse of drugs or alcohol are not classified as mental illness under the Act. Nevertheless they may lead to the development of mental conditions that may make compulsory admission necessary.

Application for admission to hospital may be made by the 'nearest relative' (who is defined under s.26). However, the 'nearest relative' may not always be readily identifiable or available, or may be too distressed to be involved in compulsory detention. It is often more practical to involve an approved social worker, who can also make the necessary application for admission.

Patients who have already been admitted to hospital or a psychiatric unit informally may require longer detention under ss.2 or 3. A patient admitted under s.2 may be detained for up to 28 days.

An order for discharge of a patient detained under s.2 may be made under s.23 by the responsible medical officer (RMO), the hospital managers or the nearest relative. The nearest relative must give at least 72 hours notice in writing to the managers, and the patient cannot be discharged if the RMO certifies that the patient is dangerous (s.25).

Where the RMO has so certified, the nearest relative may apply to the Mental Health Review Tribunal within 28 days. Where there is no nearest relative the county court may appoint another person to take over this role. The patient may also ask the hospital managers for his or her discharge. In theory, the managers could discharge the patient against the advice of the RMO. The patient may also apply to the Mental Health Review Tribunal for discharge under s.66.

Application in respect of a patient already in hospital (Section 5)

An application for admission may be made under s.5(2) by the medical practitioner in charge of the treatment of the patient where the patient is already in hospital. S.5 does not permit treatment, although emergency treatment such as sedation may be given at common law. If the patient is already receiving treatment in a psychiatric unit, a registered mental nurse can hold the patient for up to six hours under s.5(4). Ss.5(2) and 5(4) are normally used in order to allow time for formal admission and/or treatment under ss.2 and 3.

Admission for assessment in case of emergency (Section 4)

An application for emergency admission may be made by the nearest relative or an approved social worker in cases of genuine urgency on the recommendation of only one medical practitioner for a period of not exceeding 72 hours from the time of admission.

Warrant to search for and remove patients (Section 135)

Under s.135, where there is reasonable cause to suspect that a person believed to be suffering from a mental disorder has been, or is being, ill-treated, neglected or kept otherwise than under proper control or is unable to care for himself and is living alone, a warrant may be issued by a Justice of the Peace. This can authorize the removal of the patient to a place of safety by the police, in the presence of a doctor and social worker, for up to 72 hours.

Removal of mentally disordered patients found in public places by the police (Section 136)

If a police constable finds a person who appears to be suffering from a mental disorder and to be in need of immediate care, he may in the interests of that person, or for the protection of others, remove that person to a place of safety for a period of not more than 72 hours. This enables a medical examination, an interview by an approved social worker and any necessary arrangements for his care or treatment to be made.

Admission for treatment (Part V)

An application for admission for treatment may be made in the written submission of two registered practitioners who have examined the patient within 5 days of each other (one approved under the Act and the other who has preferably known the patient) on the grounds that:

a he is suffering from mental illness, severe mental impairment, psychopathic disorder or mental impairment and his mental disorder is of a nature and degree that makes it appropriate for him to receive medical treatment in a hospital; and

b in the case of psychopathic disorder or mental impairment, such treatment is likely to alleviate or prevent deterioration of his condition; and

c it is necessary for the health or safety of the patient or for the protection of other persons that he should receive such treatment and it cannot be provided unless he is detained under this section.

Applications may be made by an approved social worker or the nearest relative. However, where the application is made by a social worker it may be opposed, or prevented, by the nearest relative. Most patients treated under s.3 will have been admitted under ss.2, 4, 5 (2) or 136, although they may also be admitted directly from the community under this section. The patient may be detained for up to six months initially. Thereafter, the detention can be renewed for a further six months and then annually (s. 20).

Although psychopathic disorders are regarded as being untreatable, the 'treatability test' is satisfied if treatment either alleviates or prevents deterioration in the patient's condition. Medical treatment includes treatment of the mental disorder and its *sequelae*. Therefore, since starvation and dehydration are regarded as consequences of eating disorders such as anorexia nervosa, treatment can include the feeding of such patients (Table 6.6).

Table 6.6 Feeding of patients with eating disorders

A 37-year-old woman with anorexia was detained under s.3. The Trust sought a declaration that force-feeding would be considered medical treatment under s.63 of the Act. At a full hearing the judge held that 'force feeding will be medical treatment for the mental disorder'.
Riverside NHS Trust v. Fox (1994)
B was not suffering from anorexia nervosa, but a borderline personality disorder. She was detained under s.3 and refused to eat, and her weight fell to 32 kg. She sought and gained an injunction to prevent feeding. The Court of Appeal held that medical treatment was that which, taken as a whole, is calculated to alleviate the mental disorder. A range of acts ancillary to the core treatment fall within the scope of s.63. Hence, tube feeding constituted medical treatment, which could be carried out lawfully even without the consent of B.
B v Croydon Health Authority (1996)
The force feeding of Ian Brady, the Moors murderer, after he went on hunger strike, was held by Mr Justice Kay as 'in all respects lawful, rational and fair'. Brady was suffering from a severe personality disorder and lacked the mental capacity to refuse treatment.
R v Collins and Ashworth Hospital Authority ex parte Brady (2000)

Leave of absence from hospital (Part II)

S. 17 allows the Responsible Medical Officer (RMO) to grant leave of absence for a patient who is liable to be detained in hospital under Part II of the Act. The multidisciplinary team remains responsible for the patient's care whilst he is on leave. Leave of absence can also be revoked by the RMO for the patient's health or safety or for the protection of others.

Aftercare arrangements

S. 117 allows local health and social services to provide aftercare for patients who have ceased to be detained and leave hospital for as long as they deem the patient requires such services.

Medical treatment cannot be forced on the patient. However, re-admission may be necessary under s.3 if the patient fails to co-operate with the aftercare arrangements. The supervisor may also

Table 6.7 Mental Health (Patients in the Community Act) 1995. Supervised Discharge under s.25

Supervised discharge must be approved by: • the patient's psychiatrist • the patient's GP and • an approved social worker. There is a right of appeal to the Mental Health Tribunal by: • the patient • the nearest relative. Care in the community is the responsibility of a supervisor, who may be: • a doctor • a Community Psychiatric nurse (CPN) • an approved social worker.

convey the patient to a place where he or she is required to live or attend for treatment or training.

Some patients require a high degree of supervision if they are to live successfully in the community. These include patients at risk of personal harm or exploitation or who pose a risk to others and who will receive aftercare under s.117. Ss. 25(a) to 25(j) of the Mental Health (Patients in the Community) Act 1995 make provision for aftercare under supervision after application by the RMO to the health authority with supporting recommendations by another doctor (who will usually be the community RMO) and an approved social worker. Supervision is for six months in the first instance and then annually. Discharge from supervision for such patients is through a Mental Health Review Tribunal or the community RMO.

Discharge arrangements under the Mental Health (Patients in the Community) Act 1995 are outlined in Table 6.7.

Role of the Courts (Part III)

Psychiatrists (and others approved under s.12) may be asked to examine or admit patients by the courts, prisons or special hospitals. There is no legal obligation on the doctor to admit the patient under his or her care, but each case must be judged on its merits.

Remand for purposes of a report (section 35)

A Crown or Magistrates' Court may remand an accused person to a hospital for a report on his mental condition where the court is satisfied that the accused is suffering from a mental disorder, on the evidence of a medical practitioner, when it would be impracticable for a report to be made whilst he is on bail. The court must be satisfied that a bed will be made available within 7 days, and the accused cannot be remanded for more than 28 days at a time, or 12 weeks in all.

Remand for purposes of treatment (section 36)

Where two medical practitioners have given evidence to the effect that an accused person is suffering from mental illness or severe mental impairment of a degree that makes it appropriate for him to be admitted for medical treatment, a Crown Court may remand the accused to hospital.

S.36 only applies to an accused awaiting trial where the offence is punishable with imprisonment. As with s.35, a bed must be available within 7 days, and the accused cannot be remanded for more than 28 days at a time, or 12 weeks in all. A person remanded under s.36 is subject to the consent to treatment provisions in Part IV of the Act.

Hospital and guardianship orders (section 37)

A hospital order is an alternative to a sentence, but can only be made for offences normally punishable by imprisonment (with the exception of murder). The conditions for a hospital order are similar to those for s.3 in so far as the offender must be suffering from mental illness, mental impairment or psychopathology of a nature and degree that makes detention in hospital appropriate. In the case of mental impairment and psychopathic disorder the treatment should be likely to alleviate or prevent deterioration in the offender's condition.

The consent to treatment provisions apply as for sections 2 and 3. The duration of the order is for six months initially, but can be renewed after that time for a further six months and then annually. The RMO, but not the nearest relative, may discharge the patient. The patient or nearest relative may apply to the Mental Health Tribunal for review. The order ceases to have effect on a successful appeal.

Restriction order (section 41)

When a hospital order is made by a Crown Court, the judge may make a restriction order where it seems necessary to protect the public from serious harm. The order may be for a specific period or an unlimited time. The patient may not be granted leave, transferred or discharged without the consent of the Home Secretary.

However, the patient may apply directly to a Mental Health Tribunal, which has powers to discharge restricted patients. Such tribunals are presided over by a circuit judge or recorder.

Transfer to hospital of a sentenced prisoner (section 47)

A convicted prisoner may be transferred to a psychiatric hospital by the Home Secretary on the advice of two doctors. In addition the Home Secretary may apply a restriction order under s.49. The prisoner may apply to a Mental Health Review Tribunal within the first six months of transfer. If he is successful in the appeal and the sentence has not been completed, the patient will be ordered back to prison under s.50.

Transfer to hospital of an un-sentenced prisoner (section 48)

S.48 applies to the transfer of an un-sentenced prisoner to hospital. A restriction order (s.49) will usually be applied. The patient should normally be returned to court as soon as possible. However, if he remains unfit, a hospital order may be made in his absence and without convicting him (s.50).

Mental Health Tribunals (Part IV)

Mental Health Tribunals are independent bodies appointed by the Lord Chancellor. As judicial bodies they have power to subpoena witnesses. Membership consists of a lay member, a psychiatrist and a president, who is usually a solicitor, a barrister, or in some cases, a circuit judge or recorder.

The Mental Health Tribunal hears appeals against detention in hospital, supervised discharge or guardianship. Applications can usually be made by the patient or the nearest relative, hospital managers, the Secretary of State, and, in restricted cases, the Home Secretary. Patients may be legally represented at hearings, and may instruct an independent psychiatrist.

Consent to treatment (Part IV)

Where a patient is compulsorily detained for treatment, treatment may be given under s.63 for the mental disorder, except where such therapy requires consent and/or a second opinion (under ss.57 and 58).

> 'The consent of a patient shall not be required for any medical treatment given to him for the mental disorder from which he is suffering, not being treatment falling within ss.57 or 58 above, if the treatment is given by or under the direction of the responsible medical officer.'
>
> (s. 63)

However, as a measure of good practice, consent should be sought for all treatment even when the patient is compulsorily detained. Where a detained patient refuses to give consent, treatment may still be given in an emergency, either for mental or physical illness, under the common law principle of necessity.

Under s.57 psychosurgery and the surgical implantation of hormones to reduce male sex-drive cannot be given to either informal or detained patients without a second opinion. These two treatments require not only the patient's consent, but also the second opinion of a doctor appointed by the Mental Health Act Commission. Two other lay persons appointed by the Secretary of State must also certify that the patient has given informed consent, knowing the nature, purpose and likely effects of the treatment.

Under s.58, treatment for mental disorder may be given for the first three months of compulsory detention for treatment without the consent of the patient (except for treatment requiring both consent and a second opinion under s.57). After three months, the RMO must certify either that he has obtained the patient's informed consent (Form 38), or, where this is not possible, that a second opinion from an appointed doctor has been obtained (Form 39), unless the treatment is urgently required. Emergency treatment, which is immediately required to save the patient's life, to prevent a serious deterioration in the patient's condition, to alleviate serious suffering, or to prevent the patient from behaving violently or being a danger to himself or others is permitted under s.62. S.60 gives a statutory right for a patient to withdraw consent obtained under the provisions of s.57 and 58.

Management of the property and affairs of the patient (Part VII)

The Court of Protection is an office of the Supreme Court with powers derived from Part VII of the Mental Health Act. The Lord Chancellor appoints judges to the Court of Protection as well as a Master and other nominated officers.

The function of the Court of Protection is to manage the property and affairs of those with mental disorder who are compulsorily detained or are otherwise unable to manage their own affairs. The Court of Protection has wide powers under s.95.

The judge may, with respect to the property and affairs of a patient, do or secure the doing of all such things as appear necessary or expedient:
a for the maintenance or other benefit of the patient,
b for the maintenance or other benefit of members of the patient's family,
c for making provision for other persons or purposes for whom or which the patient might be expected to provide if he were not mentally disordered, or

d otherwise for administering the patient's affairs. Applications to the Court may be made by friends, relatives, medical authorities, solicitors and accountants.

The Court may appoint someone to act on behalf of patients. Such a person is called a receiver, and is often a relative or close friend. The Court may order an officer of the court to fulfil this role.

Legal aid/public funding is not available for proceedings. Fees are payable to the Court for its services. These are proportionate to the income of the patient and are fixed by Parliament, but can be postponed or waived in cases of hardship.

The Mental Health Commission

The Mental Health Commission is a Special Health Authority that is directly responsible to the Secretary of State and consists of lawyers, nurses, psychologists, psychiatrists, social workers and laymen.

The functions of the Commission are to:
• Appoint medical practitioners to provide second opinions in connection with the consent to treatment requirements of Part IV.
• Review the long-term treatment of detained patients.
• Visit and interview patients detained in hospitals and mental nursing homes.
• Investigate complaints in relation to detained patients.

Offences (Part IX)

The following are offences under the Mental Health Act:
• Falsification of documents
• Ill-treatment of patients who are detained or under guardianship
• Assisting patients to escape detention or custody
• Obstructing the inspection of premises, the examination of patients or the production of necessary documents or records.
However, s.139 prohibits proceedings against doctors unless an action in relation to the Act was done in bad faith or without reasonable care. Civil actions require permission of the High Court, and

Glossary of terms in the Mental Health Act 1983

Approved Social Worker (ASW)

An approved social worker is a social worker who has 'appropriate competence in dealing with persons who are suffering from mental disorder' and has been appointed by a local social services authority to fulfil this role under s.114.

Court of Protection

This is an office of the Supreme Court for the protection and management of the property and affairs of persons under a disability.

Mental Health Act Commission (MHAC)

The Mental Health Act Commission is a 'Special Health Authority'. It has powers to prepare and review a Code of Practice, including issuing guidance on specific medical treatment, and to issue Practice and Guidance Notes. It is responsible for appointing second opinion doctors. It receives reports on treatment plans and can visit hospitals and mental nursing homes, interview patients and investigate certain complaints.

Mental Health Act Managers

The Mental Health Act Managers are those who are responsible for the running of the establishment responsible for the patient. This usually means the 'hospital managers' and refers to members of the Board of the Trust. The Managers have powers under s.23 to discharge people detained under s.2, s.3. and s.37.

Mental Health Review Tribunal (MHRT)

The Mental Health Review Tribunal consists of medical, legal and lay members appointed by the Lord Chancellor to hear appeals against detention under the Act. The interested parties may have legal representation.

Nearest Relative

The Nearest Relative is the person who is nearest the top of a list of individuals set out in s.26. Where more than one person is in the same category, the Nearest Relative will be the elder relative in that category. The list, in order of preference is, husband or wife; son or daughter; father or mother; brother or sister; grandparent; grandchild; uncle or aunt; nephew or niece; or someone who is not a relative with whom the patient normally resides and has done so for at least 5 years. Where there is no Nearest Relative, or the Nearest Relative is incapable of acting by reason of mental disorder or illness, objects unreasonably or is likely to use his right to discharge the patient under s.23 without 'due regard to the welfare of the patient or the interests of the public', the Court may appoint an acting Nearest Relative.

Responsible Medical Officer (RMO)

The Responsible Medical Officer is defined in s.34 as the doctor in charge of treatment. The RMO is usually, though not necessarily, a consultant psychiatrist. A patient detained under the Act can only have one RMO at any given time.

criminal proceedings need the agreement of the Director of Public Prosecutions.

The Mental Health (Care and Treatment) (Scotland) Act 2003

The Mental Health (Care and Treatment) (Scotland) Act 2003 was passed by the Scottish Parliament in March 2003 and is expected to be fully implemented by April 2005. Advances in psychiatric treatment mean that many patients do not need to be institutionalized and can be treated under supervision in the community. The 2003 Act marks a major shift towards caring in the community and recognizes the importance of autonomy, where appropriate, and of patient advocacy for those who use mental health services. The Act incorporates many of the recommendations of the Millan Committee into mental health provision and legislation.

While there are major similarities in mental health legislation throughout the United Kingdom, the new Scottish legislation may change the situation in the next few years (Table 6.8). It will be interesting to see how changes proposed by Parliament will reflect the changes that have been passed in Scotland.

Millan Committee

The Millan Committee was set up in 1999 to review the Mental Health (Scotland) Act 1984 with particular regard to the definition of mental disorder, the criteria and procedures for detention and discharge from hospital, and the role of the Mental Welfare Commission, and to review the arrangements for sentencing and treating serious violent and sexual

Table 6.8 Summary of Mental Health (Scotland) Act 2003

> • Compulsory treatment orders permit care and treatment in hospital or in the community.
> • Creates additional safeguards in the use of certain medical treatments.
> • Makes new provisions regarding patient advocacy for those with mental disorder.
> • Identifies a 'named person' with significant rights to represent the patient's interests.
> • Places duties on local authorities to promote the well-being of those with mental disorder and to protect the vulnerable.
> • Establishes a new Mental Health Tribunal.
> • Strengthens the Mental Welfare Commission to ensure that those with mental illness and learning disabilities are adequately protected.

offenders and those with personality disorders. The Millan Report *New directions—Report of the Review of the Mental Health (Scotland) Act 1984* in January 2001 ran to over 500 pages and made over 400 recommendations. These recommendations were influential in framing the new law.

Millan Principles

The following principles were set out in the Millan Committee report and were accepted by the Scottish Executive as the basis of the new mental health legislation.

• **Non-discrimination.** Wherever possible, those with mental illness should not be discriminated against and should have the same rights and entitlements as those with other healthcare needs.

• **Equality.** The powers under the Act should be exercised without discrimination on the grounds of physical disability, age, gender, sexual orientation, language, religion, or ethnic or social origin.

• **Respect for diversity.** Patients should receive care and treatment that respects their individual qualities and abilities and diverse social, cultural and religious backgrounds.

• **Reciprocity.** Where there is an obligation for an individual to comply with a programme of treatment there should be a corresponding obligation on health and social care authorities to provide safe and appropriate services, including follow-up

arrangements after discharge from compulsory care.

• **Informal care.** Informal care should be provided wherever possible without resort to compulsion.

• **Participation.** Service users should be involved, to the extent of their capacity, in all aspects of their care. Account should be taken of their past and present wishes. Information should be provided in a way that it is likely to be understood so as to enable them to participate fully with the services being provided.

• **Respect for carers.** Those providing informal care should receive respect for their roles and experience, receive appropriate information and advice and have their views and needs taken into account.

• **Least restrictive alternative.** Care, treatment and support should be provided in the least restrictive manner. Where appropriate it should take into account the safety of others.

• **Benefit.** Any intervention under the Act should be expected to benefit the user in a way that could not be otherwise achieved than by the intervention.

• **Child welfare.** The welfare of a child with mental disorder should be paramount in any interventions under the Act.

Summary of the key changes in the Mental Health (Care and Treatment) (Scotland) Act 2003

The Act covers four important aspects of mental health legislation.

• It creates a range of duties and powers for organizations involved in mental health, including the Mental Welfare Commission and the new Mental Health Tribunal of Scotland.

• It clarifies procedures for decision-making on the compulsory treatment and/or detention of those with mental disorder.

• It amends criminal justice legislation to give courts more effective means of assessing and managing those coming before them with mental disorder.

• It creates new rights for people with mental disorder, including a right to advocacy services, and provides safeguards regarding certain treatments.

Definition of mental disorder

Mental disorder is defined as:
- mental illness;
- personality disorder; or
- learning disability, however caused or manifested.

A person is **not** mentally disordered by reason of any of the following:
- sexual orientation, sexual deviancy, transsexualism or transvestism
- dependence on, or use of, alcohol or drugs
- behaviour that causes, or may cause, harassment, alarm or distress
- acting as no prudent person would act.

Criteria for compulsory treatment

Millan tests for compulsory long-term detention

To deprive psychiatric patients of their liberty by compulsory detention and treatment is one of the most serious issues in mental health law. The Millan Committee recommended 6 tests that ought to be applied before subjecting a patient to long-term detention, which were codified in the 2003 Act (Table 6.9).

Table 6.9 The six Millan tests for compulsory detention

The six Millan tests for compulsory detention are that:
- The patient suffers from a mental disorder.
- The necessary care and treatment cannot be provided with the agreement of the patient.
- The patient's judgement is impaired to a nature or degree that justifies compulsory measures.
- The proposed treatment is likely to benefit the patient by alleviating or preventing a deterioration in the patient's mental disorder, or in associated symptoms.
- The proposed treatment is the least restrictive and invasive alternative available that is compatible with the delivery of safe and effective care.
- There is a significant risk of harm to the health or safety or welfare of the patient or a significant risk of harm to others if the treatment is not administered.

Compulsory detention and treatment under the 2003 Act

Detention may be:

- **Emergency detention for up to 72 hours (s. 36).** A medical practitioner may issue an emergency detention certificate in order to make an assessment regarding medical treatment if he is satisfied (a) that the patient has a mental disorder; and (b) that, because of the mental disorder, the patient's ability to make decisions about the provision of medical treatment is significantly impaired. The doctor must also be satisfied that if the patient were not detained in hospital there would be a significant risk (i) to the health, safety or welfare of the patient or (ii) to the safety of some other person or persons.

- **Short-term detention in hospital for up to 28 days (s. 44).** The conditions are as for emergency detention except that the purpose of short-term detention is either to determine what medical treatment should be given to the patient or to administer treatment. Emergency detention is essentially for urgent assessment, rather than for treatment, which should normally be given under the powers of short-term detention. However, treatment might still be given under common law in an emergency.

- **Compulsory Treatment Order for six months, renewable (Part VII s. 57–67).** This replaces long-term detention. Under s.57 the medical practitioners making an application must be satisfied that the patient has a mental disorder and that treatments would be likely to prevent the worsening, or alleviate the symptoms, of the disorder. There must also be a significant risk that if such treatment were not given there would be a significant risk to the health or safety of the patient or of others. The patient's ability to make treatment decisions must be significantly impaired such that the making of a compulsory treatment order is necessary. The first medical practitioner will usually be an approved psychiatrist and the second doctor will usually be the patient's GP. The requirements of the medical examination are laid out in s.58. The mental health officer has duties to identify a named person (s.59), notify the named person and Commission of the order (s.60), prepare a report (s.61) and propose a care plan (s.62). The application for a Compulsory Treatment Order must be made to the Tribunal by the mental health officer (s.63).

The Mental Health Tribunal

At present the Sheriff court authorizes long-term detention and hears appeals. The 2003 Act creates a new judicial body, the Mental Health Tribunal, to hear cases under the new Act. The Tribunal consists of three members—a legally qualified chairman, a medical practitioner experienced in mental health and a third member with knowledge of the assessment, planning and delivery of mental health services. Such a person might, for example, be a social worker, a psychiatric nurse or a voluntary sector worker. The patient may be legally represented at hearings and can present their own medical evidence. Appeals against the decisions of the Tribunal may be made to the Court of Session by the patient, the mental health officer, or the 'named person'.

Safeguards for particular treatments

Independent second opinions will be required for certain particular treatments when they are given without consent to patients subject to compulsion:
- Drugs used to reduce sexual drive
- Electro-convulsive therapy (ECT)
- Medication for mental disorder given for more than 2 months
- Medication given above recommended dosages
- Force-feeding.

Neurosurgery will require stringent safeguards:
- The patient must consent.
- Two lay persons appointed by the Mental Welfare Commission must certify that the patient can consent.
- The procedure must be approved by an experienced and independent doctor.

Rights of users and carers

The Mental Health Act introduces additional rights and safeguards for both informal users and those subject to compulsory care:
- There is a Code of Practice on the protection of the rights of informal patients.
- There is a new right for service users and their families to request an assessment of the patient's needs.
- Local Authorities and NHS Boards will be asked to make advocacy services available.
- Patients will have a right to make advance statements regarding their wishes concerning future care and treatment, which will have to be taken into account by healthcare professionals.
- Patients will have a right to a Named Person to represent their interests in Mental Health Act Proceedings. Where patients are unable to nominate such a person, the primary carer or nearest relative will take on this role.
- There will be improved procedures to intervene in cases of suspected abuse, including sexual abuse, neglect and ill treatment.

Offenders with Mental Disorder

The Act provides a wide range of means of ensuring that the offender receives the right care and treatment and that the public interest is safeguarded.

Assessment and Treatment Orders allow an accused person who is suffering from a mental disorder to be remanded to hospital for assessment or treatment. Interim Compulsion Orders allow offenders to be assessed in a hospital prior to sentencing, especially in the case of high-risk offenders. On conviction, the court may direct an offender to receive compulsory treatment using a Compulsion Order. A court may require a convicted offender to begin a prison term in hospital under a Hospital Direction

Scottish Ministers will continue to oversee the management of high-risk patients subject to restriction orders made by the criminal courts. The Mental Health Tribunal, chaired by a sheriff, will authorize discharges and transfers of restricted patients to lower levels of security.

Glossary of terms used in the Mental Health (Care and Treatment) (Scotland) Act 2003

Nurse's holding power

Power to detain a patient for two hours, plus one hour for the doctor to examine the patient.

Emergency detention

Detention for up to 72 hours.

Short-term detention

Detention for up to 28 days, with a first extension of 3 days, and a further extension of 5 days.

Compulsory Treatment Order

Initially for two six-month periods. Followed by annual renewal.

Police Place of Safety Order

Detention by police for up to 24 hours in a place of safety.

Assessment Order

Remand of an accused person suspected of mental disorder to a hospital for assessment.

Treatment Order

Remand of an accused with mental disorder to a hospital for treatment.

Compulsion Order

Sentence by a court for an offender to receive compulsory treatment.

Restriction Order

Granted by a court in conjunction with a compulsion order for those who require additional supervision within the mental health system.

Hospital Direction

Direction by a court that a prison term should commence in hospital.

Keypoints

- A knowledge of mental health legislation is essential for those working in psychiatry and anyone who may have to manage the mentally ill in an emergency.
- Compulsory detention and treatment may be required for those at risk to themselves or others by virtue of mental illness.
- Mental health legislation covers the treatment of the core mental illness and its consequences, but does not apply to other medical conditions unrelated to the mental condition.
- Legislative changes have occurred in Scotland and are proposed for England and Wales to cover compulsory care in the community.

Chapter 7

Adults with Incapacity (Scotland) Act 2000

This was the first major piece of legislation passed by the Scottish Parliament, and made substantial changes to the law in relation to the treatment of the mentally incapacitated. It lays down the principles that are to be followed by those acting on behalf of the incapacitated. The Act also provides for proxy decision-makers and for the appeals procedure to be followed in cases of disagreement regarding the medical management of patients.

Background

The Adults with Incapacity (Scotland) Act 2000 was the first Bill to be laid before the Scottish Parliament, and one of the first Acts to pass into Scottish Law in 2000. It arose from the Scottish Law Commission proposals of 1995. Similar legislation has been suggested for the Westminster Parliament. A draft Mental Incapacity Bill was published and underwent examination by a Joint Scrutiny Committee of the House of Lords and the Commons, which published its recommendations in November 2003.

The Act provides a legal framework for the management of the finances, property and personal welfare, including medical treatment, of those who lack the mental capacity to make decisions for themselves.

All decisions made on behalf of adults with impaired capacity must:
- benefit the adult;
- have due regard for the adult's wishes and feelings and those of the nearest relative, primary carer, guardian or attorney;
- restrict the adult's freedom as little as possible.

Under the Act various agencies act on behalf of the incapacitated adult:
- The Public Guardian supervises welfare attorneys and court-appointed guardians and those with access to the adult's funds (usually relatives or carers).

Table 7.1 Five overarching principles of the Adults with Incapacity (Scotland) Act 2000

Principle 1—Benefit.
Your intervention must be necessary and benefit the adult.
Principle 2—Minimum intervention
Your actions must be the minimum necessary to achieve the purpose and those least restrictive of the adult's freedom.
Principle 3—Account to be taken of the wishes of the adult
The past and present wishes and feelings of the adult must be taken into account.
Principle 4—Consultation
In deciding any intervention the responsible person must consult other relevant persons involved in the adult's care.
Principle 5—Encourage the adults to exercise their skills
The incapacitated adults should be encouraged to exercise their existing skills and develop new ones.

- Local authorities have responsibilities regarding welfare.
- The Mental Health Commission protects those who lack capacity and suffer from mental disorder. The Act allows medical treatment to safeguard or promote the physical or mental health of the adult lacking capacity. Individuals may arrange for welfare attorneys to make treatment decisions on their behalf in the event of incapacity. The Sheriff Court may also appoint guardians to make decisions on behalf of the incapacitated. The basic principles underlying the Act are outlined in Table 7.1.

The Act is divided into 7 parts:
- **Part 1.** Defines 'incapacity' and sets out the general principles regarding decision-making on behalf of the incapacitated. It lays down the roles of the Sheriff, the Mental Welfare Commission and local authorities. It creates a new office of the Public Guardian.
- **Part 2.** Provides for the registration, monitoring and supervision of attorneys with financial and welfare powers who act when the granter becomes incapacitated.
- **Part 3.** Lays down a statutory scheme to provide access to the funds held on behalf of an incapacitated adult.
- **Part 4.** Allows hospital and care home managers to manage the finances of mentally incapacitated patients or residents with appropriate safeguards.
- **Part 5.** Confers a statutory authority on medical practitioners to provide treatment to incapacitated patients and to undertake certain types of research.
- **Part 6.** Provides welfare and financial intervention orders and guardianship.
- **Part 7.** Miscellaneous provisions.

Parts 1, 2 and 5 are of particular importance to doctors, as they are concerned with the medical treatment provisions for those with incapacity.

Part 1

Part 1 provides that anything done on behalf of an incapacitated person must be done for their benefit. There is no statutory definition of 'best interests'. However, any intervention in the affairs of an adult lacking capacity must be for the benefit of the individual and be the least restrictive option in relation to their freedom.

In determining an intervention account must be taken of:
- the past and present wishes and feelings of the adult;
- the views of the nearest relative and primary carer or any other person with an interest in the welfare of the adult where it is reasonable and practicable to do so;
- the views of any welfare attorney, guardian or other person whom the Sheriff has directed should be consulted.

Definition of incapacity

Incapable means incapable, by reason of mental disorder, of:
- acting, or
- making, communicating, understanding or remembering decisions.

Incapacity is 'task-specific', so that a person may not be capable of making a major decision, but can decide simple measures. Hence a patient might lack the capacity to consent to a hip replacement, but could agree to dental treatment to relieve pain.

Definition of mental disorder

The definition of mental disorder (s.87) is the same as in s.1 of the Mental Health (Scotland) Act 1984.

'"Mental disorder" means mental illness (including personality disorder) or mental handicap, however caused or manifested; but an adult shall not be treated as suffering from mental disorder by reason only of promiscuity or other immoral conduct, sexual deviancy, dependence on alcohol or drugs, or acting as no prudent person would act' (s.87).

Judicial proceedings (Sections 2 to 5)

The Sheriff Court is the forum for dealing with various matters arising under the Act. The wide and flexible powers allow the Sheriff to:
- make rulings over and above those they have been asked to consider;
- give interim orders;
- issue directions to anyone acting under the Act such as an attorney or guardian as to how they exercise their functions;
- appoint a person to safeguard the adult's interests in any application or court proceeding;
- displace a person who would otherwise be treated as the 'Nearest Relative'.

Appeals against the Sheriff's decisions may be heard by the Court of Session, where certain matters relating to medical treatment will also be heard.

The Public Guardian

S.6 creates a new office of Public Guardian to supervise those exercising financial powers and to investigate complaints.

The Public Guardian:
- keeps registers relating to powers of attorney, use of funds, guardianship and intervention orders;
- investigates suspicious circumstances relating to the management of property or financial affairs;
- issues advice for those acting under the legislation regarding property or finances, e.g. information leaflets and other publications;
- consults with the Mental Welfare Commission and relevant local authorities about duties in which there may be common interests.

Mental welfare commission

The existence of the Mental Health Commission is governed by the Mental Health (Scotland) Act 1984. S.9 gives the Commission a range of functions, which include powers to:
- visit incapacitated adults on whose behalf others are acting;
- investigate complaints about the exercise of welfare powers by guardians, attorneys and others where the local authority has not investigated the matter satisfactorily;
- investigate suspicious circumstances, even in the absence of complaints;
- make inquiries if an adult's property or funds are at risk and, where necessary, instigate legal proceedings.

Local authorities (s.10)

S.10 of the Act sets out the role of the local authority in managing the welfare of adults without capacity. Local authority powers and responsibilities include duties:
- to monitor actions of welfare guardians;
- to consult the Public Guardian and Mental Welfare Commission where there are common concerns;
- to investigate complaints.

Part 2. Continuing powers of attorney

A power of attorney is a power conferred by a granter on another person to manage specified affairs, e.g. property and financial matters. Ordinary powers of attorney apply when the granter still has capacity. However, continuing powers of attorney continue after the granter has lost capacity to deal with the matters in question. S.15 stipulates the conditions for creating a valid continuing power of attorney. A written document is required. Oral requests would not suffice. The document conferring the power must state that it is the intention of the granter that the power should have effect in the event of their losing capacity. The power of attorney must include a certificate from a solicitor acting for the granter (or another person specified by Regulations). The solicitor (or other person acting for the adult) must certify that they have no reason to believe that the granter, who may well be a vulnerable individual by virtue of physical or mental frailty, was under any undue pressure or influence.

Exercise of welfare powers of attorney

A welfare power of attorney confers the authority to make decisions about personal welfare, including medical treatment, to another individual known as a 'welfare attorney' in the event of the granter's becoming incapacitated. Powers of attorney are only valid after registration with the Public Guardian, who must be sure that the nominated attorney is willing to accept the appointment. The conditions of the power of attorney are specified by the granter. The authority of the welfare attorney need not be affected if the granter becomes bankrupt (s.16(7)), or indeed, if the attorney becomes bankrupt. If the attorney is married to the granter, the powers cease on a decree of separation or divorce, unless the power of attorney states otherwise. If a guardian is appointed to manage the same issues as a welfare attorney, the powers of the guardian will supersede those of the attorney. Under s.20, the Sheriff has the right to make an order revoking powers of attorney and to terminate an attorney's appointment.

Attorneys are not under a statutory duty to exercise their powers. Indeed, s.17 specifically provides for attorneys to omit actions even if they are included within their authority, if they consider them unreasonable, on grounds of effort or expense, in relation to the value of the action. This protects attorneys from carrying out actions that

would be too onerous for them or of little benefit to the granter.

S.24 (4) protects those who deal with attorneys in good faith without realizing that their powers have terminated.

The role of the Welfare Attorney in medical decision-making is discussed below. However, a Welfare Attorney may not consent:

- to the granter's admission to hospital for treatment of mental disorder against their will;
- to treatment specifically restricted for the treatment of mental disorder under the 1984 Mental Health Act.

Part 5. Medical treatment and research

This is the Part of the Act that will affect medical practitioners most of all.

General authority to treat

S.47 provides authority to provide medical treatment to an adult with incapacity. Such treatment must be for the benefit of the patient (s.1). The responsible doctor may certify that the patient is incapacitated (s.47(1)). A certificate of incapacity is normally valid for one year, but this may be for a shorter period according to circumstances. During the period of validity of the certificate of incapacity, made out by the doctor with overall responsibility for the care of the adult, the responsible doctor, and those acting under his direction, have authority to do what is reasonable in the circumstances to safeguard or promote the physical or mental health of the patient. The general authority does not allow the use of force unless it is immediately necessary, and then only for the minimum time necessary (s.47(7)). Certain treatments are exempted under Part X of the 1984 Mental Health (Scotland) Act (s.48(1)). The Scottish Ministers may make regulations specifying treatment(s) that are excluded from the general authority (ss.48.(2) & (3)). Where there has been a legal challenge to the use of life-saving treatment, the general authority is restricted to treatment necessary to prevent a serious deterioration in health while the challenge is being resolved by the court. The court may withdraw the general authority for a particular treatment (s.47(10)).

Medical treatment where an attorney or guardian has been appointed

Proxy decisions may be made regarding medical treatment on behalf of the incapacitated adult by a welfare attorney, a court-appointed guardian or a person authorized to act under an intervention order, and are governed mainly by s.50. 'Medical treatment' includes any treatment designed to safeguard or promote physical or mental health.

Where the doctor primarily responsible for the care of the incapacitated adult decides to treat and the proxy refuses consent, he may request a second opinion from another doctor (known as a 'nominated medical practitioner'), who may authorize treatment. A list of independent medical practitioners who provide such second opinions is kept by the Mental Welfare Commission. The second opinion doctor must consult with the proxy. If the second opinion doctor agrees with the proxy, treatment cannot be given unless authorized by the court.

Hence, under s.50:
- The general authority does not apply where the doctor could have obtained the consent of a proxy but has failed to do so.
- Treatment may be given if a second opinion doctor certifies that in his opinion it should be given.
- Any person with an interest in the personal welfare of the adult who disagrees with the medical treatment may appeal to the Sheriff Court and thereafter to the Court of Session.
- The doctor primarily responsible for treatment may appeal to the Court of Session in the event of a disagreement with the second opinion doctor.

Research (Section 51)

Research may not be carried out except under particular circumstances and with certain safeguards. Research is not permitted where it could have been performed on those capable of giving consent. Hence any research must:

- be to obtain knowledge of the causes, diagnosis, treatment or care of the adult's incapacity;
- be likely to produce real and direct benefit to the adult;
- not proceed if the adult shows unwillingness to participate;
- have minimal risk or discomfort and be approved by the Ethics Committee;
- be undertaken with the consent of the patient's guardian, welfare attorney or nearest relative.

Part 6. Intervention and guardianship orders

S.53 gives the Sheriff the power to make one-off intervention orders that govern specific actions or decisions relating to the adult's property, financial affairs or personal welfare. Intervention and guardianship orders may involve medical treatment.

Guardianship orders may involve all aspects of the property, financial affairs, or personal welfare of the incapacitated adults. Guardianships are only appropriate where no other measures or remedies would be possible, or sufficient, in the circumstances. A guardianship order requires assessment of the adult by two medical practitioners made within 30 days of the application.

Where there is a need to assess mental disorder, one of the doctors must be approved under s.20 of the Mental Health (Scotland) Act 1984. Personal welfare applications require a report from the mental health officers of the relevant local authority regarding the appropriateness of the order. An individual applying for guardianship covering welfare matters must inform the chief social worker. The mental health officer or chief social worker is then required to make their report within 21 days for the application to proceed. The Sheriff will normally appoint a guardian for a period of 3 years, but has the discretion to make the appointment indefinite (s.58.4).

The Sheriff can appoint any individual as guardian whom he considers suitable. However, if the guardian is the chief social worker, they can only act with respect to the adult's welfare. The Sheriff is empowered to determine the suitability of the individual to act as guardian (s.59(4)). Sheriffs have powers to enforce decisions made by welfare guardians (s.70(1)) and can also order a guardian to be replaced or removed or have their powers recalled (s.71).

Non-compliance with the decisions of a guardian with welfare powers

The guardian may apply to the Sheriff for an order or warrant to enforce their decision.

Part 7. Miscellaneous provisions including duty of care

Part 7 provides for miscellaneous matters that are outlined in the Explanatory Note and are provided for under s.82 and a Code of Practice. It is important in relation to defining liability for those acting under the Act.

The Code of Practice (paragraph 5.1) indicates that under the Act attorneys, guardians and others are held at common law to owe a duty of care to the adult with incapacity. This requires the exercise of due skill and care in carrying out their functions. However, there is a limitation of liability under s.82; but even under that limitation the attorney, guardian or other appointee must act in accordance with the general principles of the Act to avoid liability. There is also a fiduciary duty under common law for the person acting on behalf of the incapacitated adult. A fiduciary duty is one based upon trust in managing the adult's financial affairs, and obliges the fiduciary to act in good faith. Those with a fiduciary duty are not allowed to enter into engagements in which they have a personal interest that conflicts with the interests of those for whom they act. Fiduciary duties also include obligations under the 'undivided loyalty rule' and the 'confidentiality rule'.

The 'undivided loyalty rule' requires that the individuals do not place themselves in a position where their duty towards one beneficiary conflicts with their duty to another. The 'confidentiality rule' requires that confidential information obtained from a beneficiary must be used for the benefit of that beneficiary and not for the attorney,

guardian or other appointee's own advantage or to benefit another.

Breach of fiduciary duty, like breach of a duty of care, normally gives rise to liability under Scottish law. However, under s.82 an attorney, guardian or person authorized under an intervention order is not liable for any breach of any duty of care or fiduciary duty if they have acted (or failed to act), reasonably and in good faith in accordance with the general principles of the Act (as set out in in s.1). However, s.83 creates a criminal offence of wilful neglect or ill-treatment of the incapacitated punishable by a fine or imprisonment.

How well is the Act working?

> **How well is the Act working?**
>
> The Public Health Division of the Scottish Executive Health Department conducted a widespread consultation process on the implementation of Part 5 of the Act, regarding medical treatment and research. The main findings were:
> - 'Incapacity' is not an all-or-none phenomenon, and should be judged in relation to particular decisions.
> - There was a need to link the Act with the Human Rights Act and to consider the role of patient advocacy.
> - There was growing concern about the resource implications of the Act.
> - Certain terms were difficult or contentious, e.g. 'benefit', 'emergency' or 'necessity'.
> - There was a concern that those with incapacity were regarded as 'mentally disordered'.
> - The boundaries between the Act and mental health legislation were often blurred.
> - There was a need to recognize the effects of physical treatment on an individual's capacity.

Glossary of terms: adults with incapacity (Scotland) act 2000

Duty of care According to the Code of Practice means 'a duty to exercise due skill and care in exercising the powers one has been given in relation to another person'.

Court Usually means the Sheriff Court. However, a few matters, such as issues relating to medical treatment, are dealt with by the Court of Session (the Supreme Court and equivalent to the English High Court in this context).

Continuing power of attorney A power of attorney granted by an individual giving particular powers as specified by the granter over their property and finances, which may be exercised in the event of the granter's becoming incapacitated.

Fiduciary duty A duty arising from a position of trust that places a special duty upon the fiduciary to act in good faith.

Guardian A person appointed by the Sheriff to act or make decisions for incapacitated adults under Part 6 of the Act.

Intervener One who acts on behalf of the incapacitated adult.

Intervention order An order made by the Sheriff under Part 6 that something should be done, or a decision made on behalf of an incapacitated adult.

Mental Welfare Commission An independent body set up by the 1984 Mental Health (Scotland) Act to protect those with mental disorder who are unable to protect themselves and their interests.

Nearest relative The person defined by the 1984 Mental Health Act as having the closest kinship with the adult. An unmarried partner or a same-sex partner for a period of more than six months may be treated as the nearest relative.

Proxy A person who is empowered to make decisions on behalf of the incapacitated. The term includes welfare attorneys, guardians and those authorized under intervention orders.

Welfare attorney An attorney appointed by an individual with particular powers as specified by the granter over their personal welfare, medical treatment, property and finances that may be exercised in the event of the granter's becoming incapacitated.

Part 4

Issues

The law in relation to abortion

'The termination of pregnancy is regulated by the law and doctors must observe the law in relation to such matters. A criminal conviction in the British Islands for termination of pregnancy in circumstances which contravene the law in itself affords grounds for a charge before the Professional Conduct Committee.'

GMC. Professional conduct and discipline: fitness to practise. February 1991

Medical students are not required to participate in terminations. Nevertheless, they will doubtless debate the ethical issues surrounding abortion during their undergraduate careers. Thirty-five years after the passing of the Abortion Act, a minority of students and doctors still find abortion deeply disturbing.

The law in relation to abortion

The law relating to abortion includes:
- the Offences Against the Person Act 1861, ss.58 and 59
- the Infant Life Preservation Act 1929
- the Abortion Act 1967
- the Human Fertilization and Embryology Act 1990 (HFEA)

'The [Abortion] Act, though it renders lawful abortions that before its enactment would have been unlawful, does not depart from the basic principle of common law as declared in *R v Bourne*, namely that the legality of an abortion depends on the opinion of the doctor. It has introduced the safeguard of two opinions: if they are formed in good faith by the time the operation is undertaken, the abortion is lawful. Thus a great deal of social responsibility is firmly placed by the law on the shoulders of the medical profession.'

Lord Justice Scarman in *R v Smith* (1973)

Offences Against the Person Act 1861

The law relating to abortion as a crime is stated in ss.58 and 59 of the Offences Against the Person Act 1861 (Table 8.1).

A woman can therefore only be guilty of procuring her own miscarriage (abortion) if she is actually 'with child'. However, anyone who administers

Table 8.1 Offences Against The Person Act 1861

> **(i) Section 58. Administering drugs or using instruments to procure abortion**
>
> 'Every woman, being with child, who, with intent to procure her own miscarriage, shall unlawfully administer to herself any poison or other noxious thing, or shall unlawfully use any instrument or other means whatsoever with the like intent, and whosoever, with intent to procure the miscarriage of any woman, whether she be or be not with child, shall unlawfully administer or cause to be taken by her any poison or other noxious thing, or shall unlawfully use any instrument or other means whatsoever with the like intent, shall be guilty of a felony, and being convicted thereof shall be liable to be kept in penal servitude for life.'
>
> **(ii) Section 59. Procuring and supplying drugs to cause abortion**
>
> 'Whosoever shall unlawfully supply or procure any poison or other noxious thing, or any instrument or thing whatsoever, knowing that the same is intended to be unlawfully used or employed with intent to procure the miscarriage of any woman, whether she be or be not with child, shall be guilty of a misdemeanour, and being convicted thereof shall be liable to be kept in penal servitude.'

Table 8.2 Infant Life Preservation Act 1929

> **Punishment for child destruction**
>
> (1) Subject as hereinafter in this subsection provided, any person who, with intent to destroy the life of a child capable of being born alive, by any wilful act causes a child to die before it has an existence independent of its mother, shall be guilty of felony, to wit, of child destruction, and shall be liable on conviction thereof on indictment to penal servitude for life: Provided that no person shall be found guilty of an offence under this section unless it is proved that the act which caused the death of the child was not done in good faith for the purpose only of preserving the life of the mother.
> (2) For the purposes of this Act, evidence that a woman had at any material time been pregnant for a period of twenty-eight weeks or more shall be *prima facie* proof that she was at that time pregnant of a child capable of being born alive.

to her, or causes her to take, any poison or noxious thing, with the intent to procure a miscarriage, whether or not she is with child, is guilty of a crime.

Infant Life (Preservation) Act 1929 (Table 8.2)

This defines the crime of child destruction, when a child who is capable of being born alive is destroyed by a wilful act, unless the act that caused the death of the child was done in good faith solely to preserve the life of the mother. The Act also states that a woman who has been pregnant for 28 weeks will be deemed to be carrying a viable child, unless it can be proved otherwise. This Act dealt with a loophole in the law, because neither s.58 nor s.59 of the Offences Against the Person Act 1861 ('OAPA') regarding miscarriage nor the law of murder, manslaughter or infanticide covered the

moment of delivery. The Infant Life Preservation Act does not apply to Scotland or Northern Ireland.

The Abortion Act 1967 (as amended) allows for abortion up to birth for severe handicap, but lowers the presumed age of viability to 24 weeks.

Abortion Act 1967 (Table 8.3)

While procured abortion remains a crime generally, the Abortion Act of 1967 decriminalized the offence provided that certain criteria are deemed to be fulfilled by two registered medical practitioners acting in good faith. In cases of emergency, the abortion may legally be performed in a place not authorized under the Act and on the opinion of only one doctor. This Act does not apply to Northern Ireland, where legalization of abortion has been resisted.

The 1967 Abortion Act (as amended by the Human Fertilization and Embryology Act 1990) defines the legal criteria for termination of pregnancy, outlines the process for notifying abortions and includes a conscience clause for those with ethical objections to participating in abortion.

There is no time-limit for the criteria in subsection (1) (b), (c) and (d). Where the 'termination is immediately necessary to save the life or to prevent grave permanent injury to the physical or mental

Table 8.3 Legal grounds for medical termination of pregnancy under the Abortion Act 1967

Legal grounds for medical termination of pregnancy
(1) Subject to the provisions of this section, a person shall not be guilty of an offence under the law relating to abortion when a pregnancy is terminated by a registered medical practitioner if two registered medical practitioners are of the opinion, formed in good faith (a) that the pregnancy has not exceeded its twenty-fourth week and that the continuance of the pregnancy would involve risk, greater than if the pregnancy were terminated, of injury to the physical or mental health of the pregnant woman or any existing children of her family; or (b) that the termination is necessary to prevent grave permanent injury to the physical or mental health of the pregnant woman; or (c) that the continuance of the pregnancy would involve risk to the life of the pregnant woman, greater than if the pregnancy were terminated; or (d) that there is a substantial risk that if the child were born it would suffer from such physical or mental abnormalities as to be seriously handicapped. (2) In determining whether the continuance of a pregnancy would involve such risk of injury to health as is mentioned in paragraph (a) or (b) of subsection (1) of this section, account may be taken of the pregnant woman's actual or reasonably foreseeable environment.

Table 8.4 Grounds for abortion on residents in England and Wales in 2002 under the Abortion Act 1967

GROUND	Number (and percentage) of abortions	
A (or with B, C or D)	118	(0.07%)
B (alone)	1,554	(0.9%)
B (with C or D)	198	(0.1%)
C (alone)	164,573	(93.7%)
D (alone or with C)	7,092	(4.04%)
E (alone)	1,770	(1.01%)
E (with A, B, C, or D)	93	(0.05%)
F or G	1	(0.00%)
Not stated	170	(0.97%)

Grounds for abortion:
A—the continuance of the pregnancy would involve risk to the physical or mental health of the mother greater than if it were terminated;
B—the termination is necessary to prevent grave permanent injury to the physical or mental health of the pregnant woman;
C—the pregnancy has not exceeded its 24th week and the continuance of the pregnancy would involve risk, greater than if the pregnancy were terminated, of injury to the physical or mental health of the woman;
D—the pregnancy has not exceeded its 24th week and the continuance of the pregnancy would involve risk, greater than if the pregnancy were terminated, of injury to the physical or mental health of any existing child(ren) of the family of the pregnant woman;
E—there is a substantial risk that if the child were born it would suffer from such physical or mental abnormalities as to be seriously handicapped;
F—in an emergency—to save the mother's life; or
G—in an emergency—to prevent grave permanent injury to the physical or mental health of the mother.
National Statistics Online

health of the pregnant woman', the pregnancy may be terminated if only one registered medical practitioner is of the opinion, formed in good faith, that an abortion is justified within the terms of the Act. The grounds for induced abortions in England and Wales in 2002 are showed in Table 8.4.

Conscientious objection

The Abortion Act has a conscience clause for those with an ethical objection to abortion, notwithstanding any duty to participate in treatment necessary to save the woman or prevent grave permanent injury to her mental or physical health. A Conscientious Clause is also incorporated into the HFEA (Table 8.5).

The legal right to conscientious objection to abortion is limited by a proximity test and does not apply to secretaries typing letters of referral for termination of pregnancy. Mrs Janaway was a medical secretary who claimed unfair dismissal for not typing a referral letter, claiming conscientious objection. The case eventually went to the House of Lords, which held that conscientious objection only applied to those directly involved in the abortion.

Table 8.5 Conscientious objection to abortion

Abortion Act 1967
Conscientious objection to participation in treatment (1) Subject to subsection (2) of this section, no person shall be under any duty, whether by contract or by any statutory or other legal requirement, to participate in any treatment authorized by this Act to which he has a conscientious objection: Provided that in any legal proceedings the burden of proof of conscientious objection shall rest on the person claiming to rely on it. (2) Nothing in subsection (1) of this section shall affect any duty to participate in treatment which is necessary to save the life or to prevent grave permanent injury to the physical or mental health of a pregnant woman. **Human Fertilization and Embryology Act 1990** **Conscientious objection** **38.**—(1) No person who has a conscientious objection to participating in any activity governed by this Act shall be under any duty, however arising, to do so. (2) In any legal proceedings the burden of proof of conscientious objection shall rest on the person claiming to rely on it.

The legality of 'medical abortions' being performed by individuals who are not 'registered medical practitioners', such as pharmacists, supplying abortifacient drugs and post-coital pills is questionable. The morning-after pill is not considered, in law, to be an abortifacient (see below). The proximity test for conscientious objection might also apply to pharmacists asked to supply or dispense abortifacient drugs. Neither the question as to whether pharmacists are covered by the Abortion Act nor whether they have rights of conscientious objection has been formally tested in the courts.

'The advent of medical termination raises the unusual position of the conscientiously objecting pharmacist who is asked to fill the necessary prescriptions; in our view, the proximity test would be satisfied, although much depends on how the relationship between the pharmaceutical and medical professions is viewed.'

Mason and McCall Smith, *Law and Medical Ethics*, 5th edn, Butterworth, London, p. 141.

Human Fertilization and Embryology Act 1990

The decriminalization of abortion signalled a major change in medical law and practice. The Abortion Act was amended in 1990 by s.37 of the HFEA so as to allow abortion up to birth where there was a risk of serious foetal handicap, or where continuance of the pregnancy would involve risk to the life of the pregnant woman, or to prevent grave permanent injury to her physical or mental health. The original Abortion Act in 1967 did not allow abortion of the viable foetus up to full term and did not permit so-called 'partial birth abortion'. This was achieved by the Human Fertilization and Embryology Act 1990 by the provision that:

'No offence under the Infant Life (Preservation) Act 1929 shall be committed by a registered medical practitioner who terminates a pregnancy in accordance with the provisions of this Act.'

The HFEA also permitted selective abortion where there was more than one foetus—a situation that may arise from the use of fertility drugs (super-ovulation) or the placement in the woman following IVF of more than one foetus so as to enhance the chances of pregnancy. Selective destruction of a viable healthy foetus could now be authorized under the amended grounds for termination of s.37(5) of the HFEA.

'(5) A woman's miscarriage (or, in the case of a woman carrying more than one foetus, her miscarriage of any foetus) is unlawfully done unless authorized by section 1 of this Act and, in the case of a woman carrying more than one foetus, anything done with intent to procure her miscarriage of any foetus is authorized by that section if

a the ground for termination of the pregnancy specified in subsection (1) (d) of that section applies in relation to any foetus and the thing is done for the purpose of procuring the miscarriage of that foetus; or
b any of the other grounds for termination of the pregnancy specified in that section applies.'

Partial-birth abortion

It comes as a surprise to many doctors and medical students that since 1990 the law allows 'abortion' up to the time of delivery in cases of severe foetal handicap even when the child would be viable. Where the foetus is killed in process of delivery, i.e. before it is fully delivered, the process has been termed 'partial-birth abortion'.

By contrast, in America, the Partial Birth Abortion Ban Act 2003 was passed by the American Senate by a majority of 64 to 34 and by the House of Representatives by 281 to 142.

Important case law on abortion

R v Bourne (1938)

This was a test case brought openly and without fee by Mr Aleck Bourne, who performed an abortion on a 14-year-old. She had been gang-raped by guardsmen in St James's Park, London. He was acquitted on the grounds that it was lawful to take into account a woman's physical and mental health needs in deciding if the doctor was acting to preserve her life. It was held that she was so traumatized by the rape that she might have committed suicide.

Mr Bourne had been a member of the Abortion Law Reform Association (ALRA). However, in 1967 Mr Bourne had become so unhappy that the landmark case in which he had been involved was being used to justify the new legislation (then the Abortion Bill) that he became a founder-member of an anti-abortion group, the Society for the Protection of Unborn Children (SPUC).

Janaway v Salford HA

Mrs Janaway, a Roman Catholic secretary, refused to type a letter of referral for abortion. It was held that typing a letter of referral did not constitute participation in abortion, and therefore Mrs Janaway was not unfairly dismissed for refusing to type the letter.

Royal College of Nursing of the United Kingdom v DHSS (1981)

Nurses in the medical team are covered by the Abortion Act, as they are acting under the instructions of a medical practitioner. They are also covered by the conscience clause.

Re F (in utero) (1988)

A local authority applied to make an unborn child a ward of court to protect it from the dangerous behaviour of the mother. The Court of Appeal rejected the application on the grounds that the court did not have the jurisdiction so to act. Furthermore, Lord Justice May held that 'to apply the principle that it is the interest of the child which is to be predominant is bound to create conflict between existing legal interests of the mother and those of the unborn child' and that 'it is most undesirable that this should occur'.

Paton v BPAS (1978) and Paton v UK (1981)

A husband sought an injunction to prevent his wife from obtaining an abortion without his consent. It was held that he had no such right and that the foetus does not have rights until it is born and has a separate existence from the mother. The decision was upheld by the European Commission of Human Rights on the basis that the abortion was performed in accordance with the mother's wishes and in order to avert a risk to her physical or mental health. However, the issue of whether the foetus would have rights and abortion would violate Article 2 (right to life) if it were viable was not decided.

C v S (1988)

In this case the unmarried father tried to prevent his former girlfriend from obtaining an abortion. The foetus at between 18 and 21 weeks showed real and discernible signs of life by virtue of a heartbeat and circulation. It was held that if the foetus was not capable of breathing even on a ventilator, it was not capable of being born alive. After the High Court and Court of Appeal had turned down the application from Mr 'C', an attempt was made to force a decision by the House of Lords, which was refused. The time from the first hearing in the High Court to an appeal and dismissal by the Court of Appeal was about 36 hours—one of the quickest in legal history. However, the effect was that the pregnant woman became so deeply affected by the case that she had the baby and gave it to Mr 'C' to look after.

Rights of the foetus

Attorney General's Reference (No 3 of 1994)

A man stabbed a woman, intending grievous bodily harm. She was between 22 and 24 weeks pregnant. Stab wounds to her lower abdomen caused injury to the foetus, and about 17 days later the woman went into premature labour. The child had an estimated 50% chance of survival, but in the event survived for 121 days before dying of broncho-pulmonary dysplasia as a result of prematurity. The man was successfully prosecuted for grievous bodily harm to the mother, and was subsequently charged with murdering the child.

The central issue was whether the crimes of murder or manslaughter can be committed where unlawful injury is deliberately inflicted

i to a child *in utero*;

ii to a mother carrying a child *in utero* where the child is subsequently born alive and enjoys an existence independent of the mother, but thereafter dies, and the injuries inflicted while *in utero* either caused or made a substantial contribution to the death.

Lord Hope held that the assault on the mother could lead to the manslaughter, but not the murder, of the child that was subsequently born prematurely but died.

'The only questions which need to be addressed are

(i) whether the act was done intentionally;

(ii) whether it was unlawful;

(iii) whether it was also dangerous because it was likely to cause harm to somebody; and

(iv) whether that unlawful and dangerous act caused the death'.

Lord Mustill discounted the view that there could be any offence against the child if it had died *in utero*, since it does not have a distinct legal personality until it is born.

'It is sufficient to say that it is established beyond doubt for the criminal law, as for the civil law, that the child *en ventre sa mère* does not have a distinct human personality, whose extinguishment gives rise to any penalties or liabilities at common law'.

Nevertheless, according to Lord Mustill the unborn cannot simply be regarded as a 'part of the mother'.

'Not only were they physically separate, but they were each unique human beings, though no doubt with many features of resemblance. . . . The mother and the foetus were two distinct organisms living symbiotically, not a single organism with two aspects. The mother's leg was part of the mother; the foetus was not.'

Lord Hope put the case for the foetus being a separate individual from the mother succinctly thus:

'The creation of an embryo from which a foetus is developed requires the bringing together of genetic material from the father as well as from the mother. The science of human fertilization and embryology has now been developed to the point where the embryo may be created outside the mother and then placed inside her as a live embryo. This practice, not now uncommon in cases of infertility, has already attracted the attention of Parliament: see the Human Fertilization and Embryology Act 1990. It serves to remind us that an embryo is in reality a separate organism from the mother from the moment of its conception. This individuality is retained by it throughout its development until it achieves an independent existence on being born. So the foetus cannot be regarded as an integral part of the mother in the sense indicated by the Court of

Appeal, notwithstanding its dependence upon the mother for its survival until birth.'

It was unanimously agreed that while the assailant intended to injure the mother, no such intention was directed at the unborn child. Therefore the criminal intention to murder the child was absent, and the case was one of manslaughter not murder. Hence, as was stated by Lord Hope:

• The mental element that is required to establish the crime of manslaughter is different from that which is required for murder.

• So far as *mens rea* for the common law crime of manslaughter is concerned, I consider that it is sufficient that at the time of the stabbing the defendant had the *mens rea* that was needed to convict him of an assault on the child's mother.

• In the present case, where there were two alleged victims—the mother who was stabbed, to whom the defendant intended to cause harm, and the child who was born later and then died, to whom no harm was intended—the question is not simply one of degree.

• The intention that must be discovered is an intention to do an act that is unlawful and dangerous.

• Manslaughter is one of those crimes in which only what is called a basic intention need be proved—that is, an intention to do the act that constitutes the crime.

St George's Healthcare NHS Trust v S (1998)

In the case of *Re: T* (1993), Lord Donaldson, MR, raised the question as to whether the need to save the life of a viable foetus might provide an exception to the need to obtain valid consent from an adult patient of sound mind:

'An adult patient who . . . suffers from no mental incapacity has an absolute right to choose whether to consent to medical treatment, to refuse it or to choose one rather than another of the treatments being offered. The only possible qualification is a case in which the choice may lead to the death of a viable foetus. That is not this case and, if and when it arises, the courts will

be faced with a novel problem of considerable legal and ethical complexity.'

Such an exceptional case arose in the case of a 36-year-old pregnant woman 'S', who was suffering from pre-eclampsia. She was advised bed-rest and induced delivery, in order to save her life and that of the unborn child. She refused. She was admitted under the Mental Health Act 1983 and subsequently transferred to St George's Hospital. The hospital authorities applied *ex parte* (that is, without notice to the woman or to any other likely or potential party) to a judge for a declaration to dispense with her refusal of treatment. This was granted and the hospital then performed a Caesarean Section and she was delivered of a baby girl.

She appealed against her detention under the Mental Health Act and for having undergone a compulsory Caesarean Section.

Her appeal was upheld by the Court of Appeal. In giving judgment Lord Justice Judge said:

'In our judgment while pregnancy increases the personal responsibilities of a woman it does not diminish her entitlement to decide whether or not to undergo medical treatment. Although human, and protected by the law in a number of different ways set out in the judgment in *Re: MB (An Adult: Medical Treatment)* [1997] 2 FCR 541, an unborn child is not a separate person from its mother. Its need for medical assistance does not prevail over her rights. She is entitled not to be forced to submit to an invasion of her body against her will, whether her own life or that of her unborn child depends on it. Her right is not reduced or diminished merely because her decision to exercise it may appear morally repugnant. The declaration in this case involved the removal of the baby from within the body of her mother under physical compulsion. Unless lawfully justified this constituted an infringement of the mother's autonomy. Of themselves the perceived needs of the foetus did not provide the necessary justification.'

Hence, as the law currently stands, a pregnant woman may refuse treatment that is necessary to save the life of her unborn child.

Judicial review of the 'Morning-After Pill' (2002)

The Society for the Protection of Unborn Children (SPUC) challenged the provision of the morning-after pill (Levonelle) through pharmacies on the grounds that it acted as an abortifacient. SPUC argued that the prescription, supply and administration of the morning-after pill by pharmacists amounted to a criminal offence under ss.58 and 59 of the Offences Against the Person Act (1861) and could only be lawful if authorized under the provisions of the Abortion Act 1967 by two registered medical practitioners.

Mr Justice Munby held:
- Prior to implantation there was not true carriage.
- The word 'miscarriage' presupposed some prior carriage.
- There could be no miscarriage if a fertilized egg was lost prior to implantation.
- Hence, miscarriage was the termination of a post-implantation pregnancy.
- The prescription, supply, administration or use of the morning-after pill accordingly did not, and could not, involve the commission of any offence under either s.58 or s.59 of the Offences Against the Person Act 1861.

Mr Justice Munby argued that since contraceptives such as the morning-after pill, the pill and the mini-pill were all used before the process of implantation had even begun, and because they could not make an implanted egg de-implant, they could not, as a matter of law, bring about a 'miscarriage'.

Congenital disabilities and 'wrongful life'

Congenital Disabilities (Civil Liability) Act 1976

The foetus has no full (nor, arguably, any) legal personality before birth. Nevertheless, under the Congenital Disabilities (Civil Liability) Act 1976, negligence towards the child *in utero* may be the subject of claims in negligence if it is subsequently born with injuries. However, the mother herself cannot be made a defendant. Moreover, a defendant will not be liable for damage if the parents were aware of the risks. Furthermore, under HFEA, a child born as a result of infertility treatment, if born disabled as a result of negligence arising in the selection, storage, or use outside the body of the embryo or gametes, is entitled to sue under the Congenital Disabilities Act.

Wrongful life, wrongful birth, wrongful pregnancy described

Wrongful life is a claim brought by the child, in effect saying that he should not have been born because he is disabled and non-existence would have saved him from such suffering.

Wrongful birth is a claim brought by the mother (or rarely the father) for the birth of a child. It arises as a result of clinical negligence in failing to identify actual or potential disablement such that the parents now have the burden of a disabled child whom they would otherwise have aborted. For the claim to succeed, the mother has to show that had she been aware of the risks she would have terminated the pregnancy.

Wrongful conception or wrongful pregnancy is where a pregnancy occurs as a result of clinical negligence, e.g. as a result of a failed sterilization.

Wrongful life

In a wrongful life claim the child is claiming that he should not have been 'allowed' to be born, i.e. that he has been harmed by being born alive with disability. The negligence occurred during, or before, pregnancy. The harm was experienced after birth.

Wrongful life claims have not been accepted by UK courts. In *McKay v Essex Area Health Authority* (1982), a woman caught rubella whilst pregnant, and the doctor did not warn the mother of the damage that might be caused to her child, which was subsequently born disabled. Had she known, she would have aborted. The case was dismissed. It was held that, although it was lawful for a doctor to advise a woman to have an abortion under the

Abortion Act 1967, the doctor had no legal obligation to the foetus to terminate its life. The child's claim that it should not have been allowed to be born alive was contrary to public policy as being a violation of the sanctity of human life. Moreover, the claim could not be recognized and enforced, since the court could not evaluate non-existence for the purpose of awarding damages.

In France, doctors were sued for failing to diagnose congenital rubella and Down's syndrome. This was deemed detrimental to antenatal care, and the law was changed (Table 8.6).

Wrongful birth

Cases have been rare in the UK, but the action is available in England and Wales. In the case of *Salih v Enfield Health Authority* (1991) the parents were awarded the basic cost of bringing up the child, not merely the difference between normality and abnormality.

In *Gregory v Pembrokeshire Health Authority* (1989) the judge found that the doctors' failure to inform of the failure of an amniocentesis was a breach of

Table 8.6 Wrongful life in France: the *Perruche* case

Nicolas Perruche was born with severe abnormalities arising from congenital rubella. In November the Cour de Cassation, France's highest court, ruled that he could sue his mother's doctors for not diagnosing his condition and offering his mother a 'therapeutic' abortion.

In July 2001 two children with Down's syndrome were awarded damages for failures to perform amniocentesis and advise termination. The French medical profession and associations for handicapped people objected to these rulings since the 'right never to have been born' would change attitudes towards handicapped people on the grounds that they should never have been allowed to be born. As a result of protests three things happened:
- Doctors refused to carry out prenatal ultrasounds.
- Practitioners' insurance premiums rose dramatically.
- Clinics stopped offering prenatal ultrasound scans.

On 10 January 2002 the French National Assembly passed the *Mattei* Bill, which effectively reversed the *Perruche* ruling.

duty of care. The action failed, however, for causation, the Plaintiff being unable to persuade the court that she would have had a second investigation had she been offered one.

Wrongful birth actions have also succeeded in Scotland; and in the case of *McLelland v Greater Glasgow Health Board* (1998), unusually, a father brought the action and succeeded.

The situation regarding abortion in Northern Ireland

Neither the Abortion Act 1967, nor s.37 of HFEA (which relates to abortion) apply to Northern Ireland. In 1945 the Criminal Justice (Northern Ireland) Act extended the terms of the Infant Life Preservation Act to Northern Ireland. Case law such as *R. v. Bourne* (1938) is also influential in determining the circumstances in which abortion is considered unlawful. The first conviction for 'child destruction' under the 1945 Act was for Colin McDonald, who stabbed his pregnant girlfriend, Michelle Kerr, 47 times in November 1997. The woman survived, but her unborn child was born dead the following day. Mr McDonald was sentenced to 22 years in prison in 2001 for child destruction and the attempted rape and murder of Michelle.

On 20 June 2000 the Northern Ireland Assembly opposed a motion extending the Abortion Act to Northern Ireland.

In July 2003 Mr Justice Kerr (now Lord Chief Justice of Northern Ireland) rejected a Judicial Review of Northern Ireland's abortion law brought by the Family Planning Association (FPA). The FPA had taken legal action on the basis that the law was unclear and in need of clarification. He said 'I'm not satisfied that it has been shown that there's any significant uncertainty among the medical community as to the principles that govern abortion.'

Conclusion

The Offences Against the Persons Act 1861 and the 1967 Abortion Act as amended provide a statutory code in relation to induced abortion. However, the Abortion Act 1967 does not apply to Northern

Ireland. The 1861 Act defines what is criminal, the 1967 Act what is lawful.

Following the Judicial Review by Mr Justice Munby, the mini-pill, oral contraceptives, the post-coital pill and the IUD are not regarded as abortifacient unless it can be shown that implantation has occurred and has been disrupted. In law, induced abortion is the deliberate termination of a pregnancy after implantation is complete. Since abortion can be procured after implantation, some forms of post-coital pill might be considered forms of 'medical abortion' and be unlawful unless covered by the Abortion Act. The grounds for abortion were extended by s.37 of the Human Fertilization and Embryology Act 1990 to include abortion up to birth (partial-birth abortion) in cases of significant foetal handicap and where there is a grave risk to the health of the mother.

Keypoints

- The Abortion Act (as amended) defines what is lawful, the Offences Against the Persons Act 1861 that which is criminal, in relation to abortion.
- The conscience clause applies to direct participation in the abortion itself.
- Nurses acting under the direction of a medical practitioner are acting within the Abortion Act.
- The Abortion Act 1967 does not extend to Northern Ireland.

Chapter 9

The ethics of abortion

Learning objectives

Core knowledge
- Arguments for and against induced abortion
- Religious and secular perspectives

Clinical applications
- Counselling women requesting abortion
- Conscientious objection

Principles
- Rights of the foetus
- Respect for pregnant women
- Abortion remains a contentious issue for some doctors, nurses and patients.
- Abortion is now regarded by many as a woman's right.
- Key issues in the controversy are the duties and responsibilities of doctors towards pregnant women and the rights and status of the human embryo.
- The issue of conscientious objection is important to those who hold that abortion means the destruction of unborn human life.

Since 1967, the law has allowed abortion for what are regarded as largely 'social', i.e. non-clinical reasons. Previously abortion had been outlawed by the General Medical Council and the Hippocratic tradition. It remains contentious for a small but significant minority of doctors, nurses and patients. However, the Abortion Act does not extend to Northern Ireland, and in Southern Ireland, where the Offences Against the Person Act 1861 still applies, abortion is still largely illegal.

The ethics of abortion may not lend itself to being an 'examination subject', and therefore we have separated it from the law on abortion. Nevertheless, the ethics of abortion will inevitably arise during the medical course and professional working life. The purpose of this chapter is therefore to raise some of these moral issues and to challenge some of the assumptions underlying the practice of abortion.

Introduction

Few issues in medicine remain as emotive or difficult as the issue of abortion. In a break with the Hippocratic tradition, abortion was legalized in this country in 1967 and in America in 1973 following the *Roe v Wade* and *Doe v Bolton* decisions of the American Supreme Court (Table 9.1).

Opinion regarding the morality of abortion remains deeply divided, and there is a significant proportion of doctors who have deeply rooted conscientious objections to abortion. The overwhelming majority of abortions are performed for 'social' reasons or are regarded a 'woman's right'. Very few abortions are recorded as having been performed for clinical reasons (see Table 8.4 of Chapter 8). However, the numbers of abortions show no sign of falling (Figure 9.1).

It has been remarked that gynaecologists do not see any inherent contradiction between inducing

Table 9.1 Landmark decisions of the Supreme Court in America in 1973

Roe v Wade

This case effectively made the right to abortion a constitutional right. It stated that a 'constitutional right to privacy' protects a woman's decision to have an abortion. Interestingly, the legal process was protracted, and 'Roe' (Norma L. McCorvey) never actually had an abortion. She has since reversed her view on abortion, and now opposes the decision in her own case.

Doe v Bolton

This case defined the health of the mother in terms of physical, emotional, psychological and familial factors, as well as the woman's age. This allowed abortion at any stage of the pregnancy. Mary Doe (Sandra Cano) was opposed to abortion in principle, but sought help from a legal aid clinic, and agreed to an affidavit that was used in the case. Money was collected for her to obtain a termination, but on the day before the scheduled abortion she ran away, and subsequently gave birth to a daughter. In 1989 she revealed the facts behind *Doe v Bolton*.

While in these two cases neither plaintiff actually had an abortion, they both later regretted their involvement in the cases that led to the legalization of abortion in America, as can be seen from the following quotations:

'I am dedicated to spending the rest of my life undoing the law that bears my name. I would like nothing more than to have this law overturned': Norma L. McCorvey ('Jane Roe' of *Roe v Wade*).

'I'm going back to court to right a wrong. Abortion has hurt millions of women and I regret my role as companion case to Roe v Wade': Sandra Cano ('Mary Doe' in *Doe v Bolton*).

---

healthy women to abort (usually with healthy foetuses) whilst at the same time regarding 'natural' miscarriage as a disease that ought to be prevented.

Few would regard induced abortion as a minor procedure. Views remain strongly polarized between those with 'pro-choice' and those with 'pro-life' perspectives.

'Pro-choice' views depend to a greater or lesser extent upon views of a woman's right to:

- privacy over her own body (a major aspect of American law in *Roe v Wade*);

- ownership of her body (of which the foetus is regarded as a part);
- self-determination or personal autonomy (a 'woman's right to choose');
- equal treatment (it is discriminatory to 'force' a woman to continue a pregnancy, since men cannot bear children).

'Pro-life' advocates, on the other hand, take the view that:

- following fertilization there exists a new human being distinct from, though clearly dependent upon, the mother. Historically, abortion was also regarded as a physical assault on the mother. In the pre-antibiotic era attempts at abortion might well have killed the woman;
- terminating the life of the foetus is thus to terminate human life, albeit in an undeveloped form.

More recently, it has been recognized that women may suffer psychological trauma as a result of abortion. In America, there has been successful litigation against doctors for failing to give adequate explanations of the psychological distress caused by abortion on the grounds that it may offend the consciences of women.

In America, claims in negligence can be filed for emotional as well as physical injury. The case of *Martinez* was a landmark for establishing a legal right to compensation for emotional injury following abortion, even without any physical injury (Table 9.2). Although an American case, it does illustrate that Post Abortion Stress is recognized as a form of post-traumatic stress disorder. It is also of interest in relation to a recent British case, in which the Rev. Joanna Jepson issued a legal challenge to a late termination performed for a cleft palate. She received the backing of the Archbishop of Canterbury, Dr Rowan Williams, who supported her efforts to stop abortions for 'trivial reasons'. (Rev. Jepson herself had been born with a cleft palate.)

Most American States have statutes that protect the rights of conscience and religion. Claims in negligence can arise in America through causing distress and violating the deeply held convictions of a patient (Table 9.2).

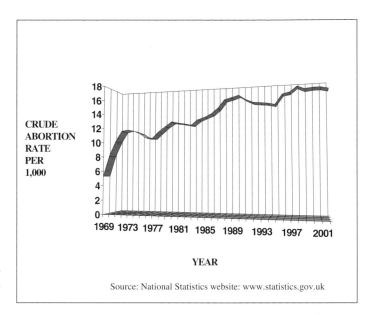

Figure 9.1 Abortion rates for England and Wales from 1969 to 2002.

Source: National Statistics website: www.statistics.gov.uk

Table 9.2 The case of Martinez v Long Island Jewish Hillside Medical Centre

> Martinez was informed that since she had taken a 'massive dose' of steroids there was a risk that her unborn child would be born handicapped with a cleft palate and severe brain damage. The child would need ventilation and then would be permanently institutionalized. Despite her strong religious beliefs, the plaintiff was persuaded to have an abortion. At the trial the plaintiff declared that she regarded abortion as wrong unless there were exceptional circumstances. In this case she had been misinformed, and there were no such exceptional circumstances. As a result she suffered five years of emotional torment and guilt. She claimed: 'Not a day goes by that I don't think about this child.'
>
> In this case it was established that:
> - There was a violation of consent because of the misrepresentation of the medical facts and of the risk to the unborn from the steroids.
> - The induced abortion plainly violated the plaintiff's conscience.
> - She would not have had the abortion if she had been properly informed of the situation.

Is induced abortion generally safer for women than delivery to term?

In 2002 there were over 175,000 abortions in England and Wales. The majority were performed for non-clinical or 'social' reasons on healthy mothers with healthy foetuses. Only a very small number of abortions were performed because of a risk to the life of the woman or to prevent grave permanent injury to her physical or mental health, or in cases of emergency (see Table 8.4 in Chapter 8).

The vast majority of induced abortions are performed on the grounds that a termination poses less of a risk to the mental or physical health of the mother than continuance of the pregnancy. Indeed, this was part of the defence in the case of *R v Smith* (1973), in which the doctor had argued that if a woman wanted her pregnancy terminated this was a powerful indication of the risk of injury to her mental health if the pregnancy was not ended (Table 9.3). It was held in that case that the doctor had not acted in good faith.

It is questionable whether a case with a similar set of facts would result in a successful prosecution today, not merely because of a change in the law but also because of a change in social values. Changes in social mores are also affected by advances in medical knowledge, and healthcare workers would be well advised to be attentive to such social changes.

There is some controversy as to the general claim (as e.g. in *R v Smith*) that abortion before 24 weeks is always safer than continuance of pregnancy.

Table 9.3 Not acting in good faith in relation to abortion certification

In 1970 a doctor undertook an operation to terminate the pregnancy of Miss Rodgers. The defendant took the view that if any girl wanted her pregnancy terminated then her wish was of itself, if not entirely sufficient, a very powerful indication of the risk of injury to her mental health if she did not have an abortion. The prosecution's case was that he had not acted in good faith. The appellant's defence was that, firstly, he had formed an honest opinion of the need for the abortion, and secondly that, in fact, at the time Miss Rodgers came to surgery, she was in process of having an inevitable abortion. The jury dismissed the latter claim.

The jury held that he had not acted in good faith. The only indications in the notes about danger to her mental or physical health were entries referring to her being 'depressed' and 'not willing to marry and depressed'. His conviction was upheld.

Lord Justice Scarman in the Court of Appeal commented:

'You have to ask yourselves, was there any balancing of the risks involved in allowing the pregnancy to continue and allowing the pregnancy to be terminated, or was this a mere routine abortion case? . . . Was a second opinion even contemplated as a necessity in this case of Miss Rodgers? If, on the very first interview when the girl was seen by the [the appellant], the very first interview he had with her, he offered to operate on her the next morning, was there any real contemplation or thought that a second opinion was necessary?'

R v Smith (1974)

There has been considerable debate about any link between induced abortion and an increased risk of breast cancer.

One meta-analysis of 28 studies of induced abortion and the incidence of breast cancer by Brind *et al*. (1996) concluded that induced abortion is 'a significant independent risk factor for breast cancer, regardless of parity or timing of abortion relative to the first term pregnancy'. However, this view has not been accepted by the Royal College of Obstetricians and Gynaecologists. The American College concluded that more recent studies argue against a causal relationship. However, full-term pregnancy appears to reduce the risk of breast cancer over a lifetime. Thus some have argued that induced abortion might have the effect of reducing this lifetime protective effect against breast cancer, which might otherwise have been gained by going to term. This finding is controversial.

However, in the short term, if abortion was generally safer for women than full-term pregnancy, one might expect a lower mortality rate in women in the year after abortion, compared to those who have continued to term or had natural miscarriages over the same 12-month period. There is little evidence on this point. However, in Finland, where there is a socialized healthcare system with accurate national statistics, the evidence seems to point, if anything, in the opposite direction — namely that the risk of suicide and all-cause mortality is greater in the year following a termination, than in the corresponding 12-month period after a miscarriage or a full-term delivery. In a study looking at pregnancy associated deaths in Finland from 1987–1994, Gissler and colleagues found that the age adjusted mortality per 100,000 was 29.4 in the 12 month period after childbirth compared with 51.3 after miscarriage and 103.2 after an abortion compared to 58.5 in non-pregnant control women between the ages of 15 and 49. The corresponding overall suicide rates were 5.9 after birth, 18.1 after miscarriage and 34.7 after abortion compared to 11.3 in the non-pregnant control patients. It has been argued that the marked increase in suicide rates in the year following induced abortion compared to full term delivery indicates either common risk factors for both abortion and suicide or harmful effects of abortion on mental health.

Similar findings of increased mortality rates in women after induced abortions and an apparent protective effect of full-term pregnancy were reported by Morgan *et al*. (*BMJ*, 1997) in South Glamorgan, who concluded that their data 'suggest that a deterioration in mental health may be a consequential side-effect of induced abortion'.

Various factors have been proposed for the increased death rate after abortion, including increased risk-taking behaviour, increased drug and alcohol abuse, increased self-destructive behaviour and domestic violence.

This research may have some legal ramifications, given that over 90% of abortions are performed on the grounds that 'the continuance of the pregnancy would involve risk, greater than if the pregnancy were terminated, of injury to the physical or mental health of the woman'. On the basis of similar research in America and Australia plaintiffs have successfully sued for a failure to warn of physical and psychological risks associated with abortion.

Abortion and Religion

Table 9.4 outlines the approaches of various religions to abortion.

Christian attitudes to abortion

While the Church of England Synod in 1983 stated that abortion was only permissible where the mother's life was in danger, individual Church members adopt a range of attitudes to abortion.

Nevertheless in November 2002 the Church of England Synod, concerned about the 500 abortions occurring in England daily, passed a motion 222 to 22 that called on the government to protect women from being coerced into abortions by providing counselling to help women keep their babies, to guarantee a woman's right to full disclosure of the risks involved and to protect those women most likely to be harmed by abortion. The current

Table 9.4 Abortion and Religion

STRONGLY PROHIBITED	ROMAN CATHOLIC Always wrong	JEHOVAH'S WITNESSES Always wrong	EVANGELICAL CHRISTIAN Many are totally opposed
VERY RESTRICTED	RUSSIAN/GREEK ORTHODOX Only justified to save mother	ORTHODOX JUDAISM Only justified to save life or prevent serious injury	HINDUISM Opposed except to save life
LIMITED	CHURCH OF ENGLAND 'Lesser evil'. Late abortions worse than early	ISLAM Sinful, worse in later pregnancy. Permitted in limited circumstances.	REFORMED JUDAISM Leaves to woman and partner. Not for 'trivial reasons'
NO WRITTEN LAW	BUDDHISM Some forbid— 'do no harm' Some allow for compassion	SIKHISM Forbidden by some allowed by others if partners agree	QUAKERS No official teaching. Reliance on individual conscience
LEFT TO INDIVIDUAL	HUMANISM Not wrong in principle	METHODIST CHURCH Permitted on compassionate grounds	

Archbishop of Canterbury, Dr Rowan Williams, is critical of current abortion services provision, and said in an interview with Roland Ashby in 1998, 'I believe abortion is taking human life and that the Church ought to declare its position on this more clearly than it often does.'

Evangelical Christians are often firmly opposed to abortion, as are Jehovah's Witnesses. Some Churches, such as the Roman Catholic Church, have clear teachings prohibiting abortion. Pope Paul IV stated (and his view has been endorsed by Pope John Paul II):

'The direct interruption of the generative process already begun and, above all, directly willed and procured abortion, even if for therapeutic reasons, are to be absolutely excluded as licit (lawful) means of regulating birth.'

Mormons are officially opposed to abortion except when the pregnancy results from incest or rape, when the life or health of the mother would be seriously jeopardized or when the foetus has serious defects that would not allow it to survive beyond birth.

Islam and abortion

In Islam, all human life is regarded as sacred from conception to natural death. Islamic law prescribes clear punishments for anyone performing or assisting at abortion. *Al Gurrah* (blood money) is payable if the baby is aborted dead, and full *diyyah* (compensation) is payable if the baby is aborted live.

On the other hand, there is a difference of opinion among the scholars about whether abortion is permitted during the first four months of pregnancy, and for what reasons. Few scholars consider it better than detestable (*makruh*), that is, better to avoid but not punishable if done. The majority of scholars hold that as a general rule it is forbidden, but that there may be specific exemptions or concessions under the law. They also differ on how extensive those exemptions are.

Various Islamic scholars, e.g. Ibn Tayamiyah, Imam Al Ghazzali and Imam Malik, have rejected abortion altogether. Al Ghazzali taught that it is a crime to disturb the fertilized egg and that the crime becomes worse as pregnancy progresses. There is nothing in the Qur'an that allows abortion, and these scholars hold that the Qu'ran does not permit it. They cite, among other verses:

'Whoever kills a human being [a soul], unless it be for murder or corruption on earth, it is as though he had killed all mankind, and whoever saves a life it is as though he had saved the life of all mankind.'

(Qur'an, Ch. 5, v. 31)

Overall, one can say that abortion is permissible in limited circumstances during the first four months, but that the restrictions become greater as the foetus develops and comes closer to ensoulment, which is reckoned to occur at about the fourth month. However, there are varying schools of thought, and healthcare workers will need to be sensitive to that fact.

Hinduism and abortion

Hindu scriptures and tradition have condemned abortion, except where the mother's life is in danger. The foetus is a living person deserving protection according to that tradition. Abortion thwarts a soul in its progress towards God. Hindu scripture refers to abortion as *garha-batta* (womb killing) and *bhroona hathya* (killing the undeveloped soul). India's greatest advocate of non-violence, Mahatma Ghandhi, wrote in *All men are Brothers, Autobiographical Reflections*: 'It seems to me clear as daylight that abortion would be a crime.'

Buddhism and abortion

In Buddhism abortion is also viewed negatively. Abortion is a violation of the First Precept against taking life, particularly the karmically advanced life of a developing human being. The prohibition against taking life is part of a reverence for life that is one of Buddhism's three basic goods — 'life, wisdom and friendship'. Nevertheless, there is no overriding ethical authority in Buddhism, and individuals must make up their own minds. Hence the Dalai Lama in an interview in 1993 reported in the *New York Times* stated that 'Of course, abortion, from a Buddhist viewpoint, is an act of killing and is negative, generally speaking. But it depends on the circumstances. If the unborn child will be retarded or if the birth will create serious problems for the parent, these are cases where there can be an exception. I think abortion should be approved or disapproved according to each circumstance.'

Sikhism and Bahaism and abortion

While not absolutely prohibited, abortion is generally unacceptable in Sikhism and Bahaism. In Sikhism abortion is taboo, as it interferes with the creative work of God. Once conception has occurred deliberate abortion or procurement of miscarriage is forbidden. Bahais believe that the soul is associated with the body at the time of conception, and the deliberate taking of human life is generally not permitted. For this reason the intra-uterine device, because of its abortifacient nature, is unlikely to be chosen as a form of birth control. Abortion merely to prevent the birth of an unwanted child is also forbidden.

Relevance to healthcare workers

It can be seen that the subject of abortion remains a delicate one, and one that can be difficult for healthcare workers where there are religious or other conscientious objections to the procedure.

In order to avoid potential problems it will be helpful for healthcare workers to be aware of the varying types of religious and other conscientious objections to the procedure, so as to avoid any potential ethical or legal problems with patients who might hold such views.

Conscientious objection to abortion

Some healthcare professionals themselves object to the procedure and believe that abortion involves the killing of an innocent human being in the womb. They will not wish to be involved in abortion, and may claim a right of conscientious objection.

The BMA amended its guidance to take into account a resolution passed by the Annual General Meeting in 1999 that abhorred harassment or discrimination against doctors 'who conscientiously object to participation in terminations of pregnancy. Doctors with a conscientious objection must now make their views known to patients seeking terminations and should ensure that the treatment or advice they provide is not affected by their personal views.'

The Abortion Law Reform Association (ALRA) was set up in 1936 specifically to campaign for legal abortion. In 1998 ALRA conducted a survey in which it found that a significant proportion of trainees were opting out of training in abortion (Table 9.5).

Thirty-six years after the passage of the Abortion Act there also remains disquiet on the issue of abortion amongst GPs (Table 9.6).

Referrals for abortion and conscientious objection

The issue of referral for abortion is a problem for those with a fundamental objection to abortion. Those with an objection to the procedure, particularly those who believe that termination of human life is involved, do not always feel comfortable about referring the patient to another doctor who does not object. However, in his judgment in the House of Lords in *Janaway*, Lord Keith of Kinkel stated

Table 9.5 ALRA Survey of attitudes and experience of abortion amongst trainees in gynaecology

ALRA carried out two surveys—the first survey was of all consultant obstetricians and gynaecologists responsible for training in the UK (300) and the second was of a sample of trainees (201 registrars and house officers). They found that:
- one-third of trainees had not trained in abortion techniques and a similar percentage had a conscientious objection to abortion; and
- three out of ten consultants said they had problems in recruiting sufficient juniors to carry out abortions, and four out of ten felt that the situation would get worse.

Table 9.6 GP attitudes to abortion

In a GP survey conducted by Marie Stopes International in 1999:
- 18% of doctors were broadly anti-abortion;
- one in five (19.8%) felt that the current law was being interpreted too liberally and should be amended to restrict access to abortion;
- 40% disagreed with the view that the Abortion Act should be altered to allow a woman a right to choose abortion in the first 14 weeks of pregnancy after consultation with a doctor;
- 46% of GPs felt that the woman alone should decide in the first trimester.

'it does not appear whether or not there are any circumstances under which a doctor might be under any legal duty to sign a green form so as to place in difficulties one who had a conscientious objection to so doing. The fact that during the 20 years that the Act of 1967 has been in force no problem seems to have surfaced in this connection, may indicate that in practice none exists.'

The National Institute of Clinical Excellence (NICE) has published guidelines for antenatal care that include universal screening for Down's syndrome, although 'a woman's right to accept or decline the test should be made clear'.

In order to avoid problems compromising those with conscientious objections to abortion, it has been suggested that they declare their objections so that they are not directly involved in counselling women who might be seeking abortion. This should not however prevent women who nevertheless wish to consult doctors with a conscientious objection to abortion from being permitted to do so.

The General Medical Council (GMC) in its booklet *Good Medical Practice* states that general practitioners' views about a patient's lifestyle or beliefs must not prejudice the treatment they provide or arrange. If doctors feel that their beliefs might affect the treatment, this must be explained to the patient, who should be told of her right to see another doctor.

Professor Mike Pringle, chairman of the Royal College of General Practitioners, (RCGP) has said:

'We support a woman's right to make considered decisions within the limits of the law and believe GPs should have the right to choose their stance as long as it does not affect a woman's right to choose or access services.'

Ethical issues in 'wrongful life' and 'diminished life' claims

Wrongful life and diminished life claims might be thought to arise because of a perceived duty of the doctor to:
- ensure physically and mentally healthy offspring;
- report abnormalities affecting the child *in utero* during screening programmes or detected routinely, e.g. during a prenatal scan;
- warn of possible side-effects from medication or investigations, e.g. anti-epileptic medication or radiation risks from radiology;
- warn of potential risks to the foetus due to medical conditions arising in pregnancy, e.g. maternal rubella.

There are a number of congenital conditions that can give rise to pain, suffering or disability in later life. Might there be a duty of care to prevent such disabilities, even if this inevitably meant a referral for abortion? Professor Amos Shapira (1998) has argued that

'The plaintiff's defective life (where healthy life was never an option) constitutes a compensatable injury. A sufficient causal link may exist between the plaintiff's injury and the defendant's breach of duty of due professional care, and an appropriate measure of damages can be allocated to the disabled newborn.'

He further asserts that the genetic counsellor owes a duty of care to the newborn and that the birth of a defective foetus should be avoided or else the mother should be advised of the risks. He felt that there was no inherent injustice in holding counsellors liable for negligence in such circumstances, and that there may be a public interest in so doing.

However, there are competing arguments against wrongful life claims, raising such issues as:
- Is there a right not to be born?
- Is the child really the 'victim' of negligence,

since without the 'negligence' it would never have been born?

• Wrongful life claims discriminate against the disabled and affect the view that others take of those who are disabled.

• Wrongful life claims challenge the 'sanctity of life' principle and the idea that all human beings have a fundamental right to life (see Article 2 of the European Convention).

• If abortion is allowable for disability in the un-born, why not euthanasia and physician-assisted suicide after birth for the same reasons?

• The presumption that a disabled life is not worth living and that the disabled would be better off dead is inherently unprovable as a matter of law. The dead cannot testify to this hypothesis.

• Is the disability of a child an addressable harm if it has not arisen through anyone's fault?

• Compensation is usually given to restore the status quo before the injury. However, in these cases the *status quo ante* would be a state of non-existence for the individual. To compare impaired existence with non-existence is not logical or justiciable, and could not be the subject of a mean-ingful judicial decision.

• If, in the evaluation for purposes of compensa-tion, an impaired life is balanced against an unim-paired life, this would not be a fair comparison if there was never any prospect of an unimpaired life, e.g. if the child had Down's syndrome.

• If wrongful life claims can be made against doc-tors, then why not against the parents?

• If the child has not been harmed, disadvantaged or wronged except through 'natural causes', why should it be compensated? Patients suffering from disease arising through no one's fault do not receive damages simply because they suffer the misfortune of being ill.

• A congenitally disabled child may suffer harm, but has not necessarily been wronged.

British courts have not been attracted to 'wrongful life' claims (brought by the child) largely for these reasons. 'Wrongful birth' claims (brought by one or both of the parents), however, have been met with some success, although many of the above objections have been associated with that class of claims also, and may continue to persuade the courts to continue to adopt a restrictive view of such actions.

Abortion and discrimination—is it an issue for medical students?

A concern about discrimination in the admission of students to medical school was recently ex-pressed in Parliament. However, discrimination was strenuously denied by the Chairman of the Council of Heads of Medical Schools, Professor Boyd, who denied allegations that medical schools were restricting the admission of Muslim students after complaints that they are forcing doctors to abandon the teaching of certain subjects on religious grounds.

Conclusion

Approximately 500 abortions are performed each day in Britain, making this one of the most fre-quently performed surgical operations. Neverthe-less, the indications in over 90% of cases are 'social'. Indeed, some argue that the termination of pregnancy is a decision for the woman, and no one else. However, it is important to consider the implications of surgery performed primarily for social or psychological reasons.

It is difficult to obtain comprehensive long-term data on the physical and psychological effects of induced abortion. The available evidence does not seem very encouraging. Indeed, a Commission of Inquiry into the operation and consequences of the Abortion Act on the physical and psycho-social effects of Abortion, chaired by Lord Rawlinson QC, concluded that the

'Psychological effects [of induced abortion] may be short-term or long-term. Acute short-term effects requiring hospitalisation are low, but given the large number of abortions carried out annually, do result in significant numbers of new cases every year. Less acute effects are under-estimated due to very high attrition rates in surveys attempting to investigate the effects of abortion at periods of longer than a few months after the event.'

The conscience clause applies to actual participation in the abortion itself. Those with conscientious objections have been advised to indicate their views to employers, trainers and patients. A growth in litigation for 'wrongful birth' of disabled foetuses may cause those with conscientious objections to distance themselves from women seeking abortion or from being involved in screening programmes; and healthcare workers need to be aware of developments in this area if they are likely to come across the issue in their own careers.

Keypoints

- Abortion remains a contentious issue for some doctors, nurses and patients.
- Abortion is now regarded by many as a woman's right.
- Key issues in the controversy are the duties and responsibilities of doctors towards pregnant women and the rights and status of the human embryo.
- The issue of conscientious objection is important to those who hold that abortion means the termination of unborn human life.

Chapter 10

Reproductive technology and surrogacy

Learning objectives

Core knowledge
1 Human Fertilization and Embryology Act 1990
2 Role of Human Embryology and Fertilization Authority to license research and treatment

Clinical applications
1 Artificial insemination
2 *In vitro* fertilization

Background principles and case law
1 Ethics of embryo research and human cloning
2 Ethics of pre-implantation genetic diagnosis
3 Use of foetal tissue for transplantation
4 Rights and duties of genetic parents in reproductive technology
5 Right to know one's genetic identity and parentage
6 Confidentiality of gamete donors
7 Moral status of the human embryo
8 *Hashmi*, *Blood* and *Whitaker* cases

Introduction

Up to one in six couples are infertile, and many seek medical help with assisted conception techniques—mainly *in vitro* fertilization and donor insemination (Table 10.1). These techniques and research into reproductive technology can only be provided under licence from the Human Fertilization and Embryology Authority, which was set up under the Human Fertilization and Embryology Act 1990.

A wide variety of artificial reproductive techniques are now available, including artificial insemination by husband or donor, *in vitro* fertilization with or without sperm or egg donation, embryo donation, gamete intra-fallopian transfer (GIFT) using the couple's own or donated sperm or eggs, and intra-cytoplasmic sperm injection (ICSI).

Human Fertilization and Embryology Act 1990

Definitions

Embryo

This is defined in s.1.

'1 (a) embryo means a live human embryo where fertilization is complete, and references to an embryo include an egg in the process of fertilization, and, for this purpose, fertilization is not complete until the appearance of a two cell zygote'.

Mother

This is defined in s.27 in relation to the gestational mother—who is not necessarily the genetic mother.

Table 10.1 Assisted reproduction statistics

General statistics on assisted reproduction
1 One in six couples will have fertility problems.
2 IVF accounts for about 1% of all births in the UK.
3 Since the first IVF baby Louise Brown was born in 1978, there have been over 68,000 children born though IVF in the UK.
4 Treatment costs range from £2,000 to £4,000, with drugs costing up to an additional £1,000.
5 Causes of infertility: female factors 40%, male 30%. The remaining 30% is due to infertility in both partners or is unexplained.
6 Success rates:
• Overall success (live births) for all IVF patients was about 22%.
• 25% in those under 38 years.
• Overall live birth rate for patients treated with donor insemination was about 11%.

Source: HFEA. Statistics are for April 2000 to March 2001

'27 (1) The woman who is carrying or has carried a child as a result of the placing in her of an embryo or of sperm and eggs, and no other woman, is to be treated as the mother of the child.'

Father

A 'father' is defined in s.28. The definition of 'father' is rather more complicated than that of 'mother', and the concept can be defined in a number of ways, although a child can only have one father.

1 As the spouse of the mother and donor of the sperm.

2 If the mother was party to a marriage, and her spouse, though not the genetic father, consented to 'the placing in her of the embryo or the sperm and eggs or to her insemination, then he shall be regarded as the father of the child'.

3 As the father recognized by virtue of the rules of common law or other rule of law.

4 As the father by virtue of the adoption of the child.

However, an anonymous sperm donor would not be held as the father (s.28.6(a)).

Some of the complexities of defining fatherhood

Table 10.2 Fatherhood and IVF

Dame Elizabeth Butler Sloss, President of the Family Division, ruled that the black genetic father (Mr B) of mixed-race twins born to a white couple after an IVF mix-up is also their legal father. Custody had been given to the white couple (Mr and Mrs A). The ruling means that Mr B could have rights over the children's upbringing and Mr A would have to apply for adoption if he wished to become their legal father.
Leeds Teaching Hospitals NHS Trust v A & B & HFEA (2003)
In a separate case, a mother conceived a girl through IVF with the consent of her former partner. Initial attempts at IVF failed, but the woman returned a year later to use the stored embryos without informing the clinic that she had separated from her partner. The man claimed that he was the legal father, since he had signed the original consent form. In the Court of Appeal, Lady Justice Hale ruled against him. She held that 'fatherhood' as defined by the HFE Act did not begin until the embryo is placed inside the woman. In this case, since the couple were no longer together when this occurred, he is not the father.
In re R (a child) (2003)

in relation to IVF are illustrated in Tables 10.2 and 10.3.

Parental orders in favour of gamete donors

S.30 allows the court to make 'an order providing for a child to be treated in law as the child of the parties of the marriage (referred to in this section as 'the husband' and 'the wife') if:

a the child has been carried by a woman other than the wife as the result of the placing in her of an embryo or sperm and eggs or her artificial insemination,

b the gametes of the husband or the wife, or both, were used to bring about the creation of the embryo'.

However, there are conditions to the child's being accepted as a party to the marriage:

i The order must be made within 6 months of the birth of the child.

ii The child's home must be with the husband and

Table 10.3 Posthumous conception and the Deceased Fathers Act 2003

Mr Stephen Blood died of bacterial meningitis in 1995, but he and his wife had been trying for a family for some time. While he was in a coma Mrs Diane Blood persuaded doctors to obtain some of his sperm so that she would be able to conceive through artificial insemination.

The Court of Appeal held that the use of the sperm in the UK would be unlawful, as it had been obtained without written consent, and the HFEA had no discretion to allow its use in the UK. However, under European Community law Mrs Blood had a right to receive treatment abroad. In 1997 the HFEA issued a Special Direction permitting the export of sperm to the Centre of Reproductive Medicine in Brussels. Mrs Blood has since conceived two sons, Liam and Joel.

Mrs Blood continued her fight to gain recognition of Stephen as the legal father of her boys. Her campaign led to the introduction of the Human Fertilization and Embryology (Deceased Fathers) Act 2003, which allows a man to be recorded as the father on the birth certificate when a child is born as a result of fertility treatment after his death.

R v Human Fertilization and Embryology Authority ex.p. Blood (1997)

wife, who must be domiciled in the United Kingdom, Channel Islands or Isle of Man.

iii The husband and wife must be over 18 years.

iv The court must be satisfied that the father of the child (including any man defined as 'father' under s.28) and the woman who carried the child have freely and unconditionally agreed to the making of the order—unless such a person cannot be found or is incapable of giving agreement. (The agreement of the woman who carried the child is regarded as being ineffective if given less than 6 weeks after the birth.)

v No money or other benefit (other than reasonable expenses) must have been given or received by the husband or wife.

Anonymity of gamete donors

The ability to discover one's genetic heritage and parentage is seen by some as a human rights issue.

At present the HFEA must keep records of gamete donors, so that future children may have limited information about their genetic parents. However, the HFEA cannot provide identifying information to children of assisted reproduction.

Removal of donor anonymity would mean the prospect of a 'knock on the door' by the offspring of donors. Government proposals to remove gamete donor anonymity would give children the legal right to trace their genetic parents, but were rejected by the BMA for fear of reducing donations. However, when donor anonymity was removed in Scandinavian countries there was an initial drop in donations followed by a return to normal levels.

Adam and Jo Rose, a brother and sister whose biological father is an unknown sperm donor, claimed in the High Court that the present law banning disclosure of information about sperm donors breaches Article 8 of the Human Rights Convention. The action is being supported by the civil rights group, Liberty. It appears that the government has conceded the principle, but is not willing to remove anonymity retrospectively.

HFEA guidance on egg giving and sharing

The HFEA guidance on egg giving and sharing is shown in Table 10.4.

There is a legal ban on the use of foetal ovarian tissue as a source of eggs for reproductive purposes (Table 10.5).

The Human Fertilization and Embryology Authority

The Human Fertilization and Embryology Authority was established under s.5 of the 1990 Act and acts as a licensing authority for the provision of reproductive treatment services and the storage of embryos and gametes and for embryo research.

Licences for treatment (Schedule 2)

'Treatment services' are defined as 'medical, surgical or obstetrical services for the purpose of assisting women to carry children'. However, once an

Table 10.4 HFEA guidance: egg giving and sharing

Egg sharing involves collecting additional eggs from one IVF cycle for donation. In return the woman receives IVF treatment at a reduced rate. Altruistic donation is where a woman donates all her eggs without undergoing infertility treatment herself.

Egg giving involves a woman's undergoing two treatment cycles, in which one treatment cycle is used to provide eggs for donation and the other is used for IVF treatment for the woman at reduced cost. Egg giving involves a second treatment cycle, with an additional risk of ovarian hyper-stimulation syndrome (OHSS).

In December 2003 egg giving was banned by the HFEA. Suzi Leather, Chair of the HFEA, said:

'There is a shortage of donor eggs in the UK and the distress of women who face long waiting lists for treatment is very real. But the HFEA cannot allow clinics to offer a treatment where a woman, for no other reason than financial inducement, subjects herself to an unnecessary and possibly risky procedure.'

In October 2003, the HFEA confirmed advice issued in 1994 that it would not allow the donation of eggs from deceased women.

Table 10.5 HFEA confirms the legal position on the use of foetal ovarian tissue (July 2003)

The Human Fertilization and Embryology Authority (HFEA) have confirmed that the use of foetal ovarian tissue in fertility treatment is currently banned in the UK.

The Criminal Justice and Public Order Act 1994 amended the Human Fertilization and Embryology Act 1990 to include a ban on the use of foetal ovarian tissue in fertility treatment.

The HFEA Chair, Suzi Leather, said:

'The use of foetal ovarian tissue raises difficult social, ethical, legal and scientific concerns. After the HFEA public consultation in 1994, it was clear that in the current social climate it would be difficult for any child to come to terms with being created from aborted foetuses.'

The HFEA has not banned the use of foetal material to produce eggs for research purposes if fully informed consent is given, but the HFEA has not yet granted any licences for this research.

Table 10.6 Consent required for use of stored embryos from both partners

In a High Court Decision, Natallie Evans and Lorraine Hadley were prevented from using their stored frozen embryos without the consent of their former partners. Ms Evans had six stored embryos created with her then boyfriend's sperm after it was discovered that her ovaries were pre-cancerous and had to be removed. Ms Hadley had two stored embryos, which her husband refused to allow to be used after the end of their marriage.

Mr Justice Wall held that, while he had sympathy with the women, he could not override the law. Schedule 3 of the Human Fertilization and Embryology Act 1990 (Schedule 3) states:

'An embryo the creation of which was brought about *in vitro* must not be kept in storage unless there is an effective consent, by each person whose gametes were used to bring about the creation of the embryo, to the storage of the embryo and the embryo is stored in accordance with those consents.'

Suzi Leather, the Chair of the HFEA, commented:

'It is very important that people who are going for fertility treatment understand the law which governs what happens to embryos in storage. Both parties must give their consent not only for embryos to be created but also to be stored. If one partner withdraws their consent the embryos cannot be stored any longer.'

embryo is produced *in vitro* it is legally necessary to have the consent of both partners for implantation to proceed (Table 10.6).

Licences may 'authorise any of the following in the course of providing treatment services':

a Bringing about the creation of embryos *in vitro*;

b Keeping embryos;

c Using gametes;

d Practices designed to secure that embryos are in a suitable condition to be placed in a woman or to determine whether embryos are suitable for that purpose;

e Placing any embryo in a woman;

f Mixing sperm with the egg of a hamster, or other animal specified in directions, for the purpose of testing the fertility or normality of the sperm;

g Any other practices as may be specified in, or determined in accordance with, regulations.

However, a licence cannot be granted for 'any activity unless it appears to the Authority to be necessary or desirable for the purpose of providing treatment services'. Furthermore, a licence 'cannot authorise altering the genetic structure of any cell while it forms part of an embryo'.

As a condition of a licence for treatment account must be taken 'of the welfare of any child who may be born as a result of the treatment (including the need of that child for a father), and of any other child who may be affected by the birth' (s.13(5)).

Licences for research

A licence may authorize 'bringing about the creation of embryos *in vitro* and the keeping or using of embryos for the purposes of a project of research.' An embryo produced by cell nuclear replacement (CNR) is regarded as an embryo under the Act following a decision by the House of Lords in March 2003 (Table 10.7).

Licences for research are limited to specific purposes, namely:

1 promoting advances in the treatment of infertility;

2 promoting knowledge about the causes of congenital disease;

3 increasing knowledge about the causes of miscarriages;

4 developing more effective techniques of contraception; or

5 developing methods for detecting the presence of gene or chromosome abnormalities in embryos before implantation, or for such other purposes as may be specified in regulations.

However, under s.3(3):

'purposes may only be so specified (under (e)) with a view to the authorization of projects of research which increase knowledge about the creation and development of embryos, or about disease, or enable such knowledge to be applied'.

Furthermore,

'no licence shall be granted unless the Authority

Table 10.7 House of Lords confirm use of cloned human embryos for research

The Pro-Life Alliance had previously argued in court that the HFE Authority was not entitled to regulate the use of cloned embryos. The central issue was whether a clone produced by cell nuclear replacement (CNR) was an embryo within the terms of the HFE Act 1990. The Alliance had argued that a human clone was not an embryo under the Act, since it had not been produced as a result of fertilization of an egg by a sperm, i.e. they were not 'cells having undergone fertilization'.

The House of Lords held that embryos created outside the body came within the regulatory powers of the HFE Act 1990 regardless of how they were created. This decision enables HFEA to license research projects on cloned embryos and following parthenogenesis in which unfertilized eggs are induced to divide after chemical or electrical stimulation.

R v Secretary of State for Health ex p. Quintavalle (on behalf of Pro-Life Alliance) (2003)

One of the first such licences for research on cloned embryos was granted to the Roslin Institute in Edinburgh—the home of Dolly the cloned sheep.

The Human Reproductive Cloning Act 2001 banned reproductive cloning, making it an offence to place in a woman a human embryo created other than by fertilization of egg and sperm.

is satisfied that any proposed use of embryos is necessary for the purposes of the research'.

The HFE Act therefore permits the creation of human embryos specifically for research, as well as the use of 'spare' embryos for research purposes. However, according to s.3 no living embryo can be kept or used after the appearance of the primitive streak or more than 14 days after fertilization, not counting any time of storage. The HFE Act therefore effectively authorizes both destructive embryonic research and also the destruction of a viable foetus if it was likely to be born seriously disabled or threatened the life of the mother, as was seen in the previous chapter.

Should 'designer babies' be allowed?

The possibility of pre-implantation diagnosis and sex selection has raised a number of complex issues. Should pre-implantation genetic diagnosis

Table 10.8 The Hashmi, Whitaker and Masterton cases

The Hashmi Case

In December 2001 the HFE Authority gave permission for Raj and Shahana Hashmi to select an embryo and produce a sibling who would act as a suitable donor to provide umbilical cord cells for their four-year-old son Zain, who suffers from ß-thalassaemia. A case was brought against the Authority by Josephine, Countess Quintavalle of CORE (Comment on Reproductive Ethics) on the grounds that the HFE Authority had acted beyond its powers. She won in the High Court, but the decision of Mr Justice Kay was overturned by the Court of Appeal in April 2003.

R (Quintavalle) v HFEA (2003)

The decision in the case of the Whitakers

In contrast to the Hashmi case, the HFE Authority had ruled against tissue-typing for the purpose of selecting a donor for Charlie, the son of Michelle and Jayson Whitaker, who suffers from Diamond-Blackfan anaemia. The HFE Authority had ruled against embryo selection on the grounds that it would not directly benefit the embryo. As a result the Whitakers had a genetically selected child in a Chicago clinic. The child Jamie was born in Sheffield in June 2003.

The decision in the case of the Mastertons

Alan and Louise Masterton lost their daughter Nicole in a bonfire accident. They have four sons and wanted to have another baby girl through IVF and sex selection by pre-implantation genetic diagnosis (PGD). The Mastertons argued that they were not seeking a 'designer baby', but that they had a need to restore their family's 'female dimension' for the sake of their psychological health. The HFE Authority refused permission. HFE Authority guidelines prevent choosing a baby's sex except for exceptional medical reasons, e.g. haemophilia or muscular dystrophy.

---

be permitted where there is a risk of severe genetic disease? Should children be produced and selected for use as potential donors for siblings? Should parents be allowed to select the sex of their children? Three important cases have arisen recently (Table 10.8).

Surrogacy

Surrogacy arrangements are not legally recognized in Britain. The Human Fertilization and Embry-ology Act 1990 inserted a new section, s.1(a), into the Surrogacy Arrangements Act of 1985:

'1 (a) No surrogacy arrangement is enforceable by or against any persons making it.'

'Surrogacy arrangements' refers to arrangements as defined by the Surrogacy Arrangements Act 1985, and does not include agreements made after the child is conceived and where it is intended that the child shall be handed over to the surrogate mother.

However, an offence might be committed under s.57 of the Adoption Act 1976 if the commissioning couple were to intend adoption of the child after birth and there had been any payment to pave the way for a future adoption.

The HFE Authority in its Code of Practice in 1998 regarded surrogacy only as a means of last resort:

'The application of assisted conception techniques to initiate a surrogate pregnancy should only be considered where it is physically impossible or highly undesirable for medical reasons for the commissioning mother to carry the child.'

The Surrogacy Arrangements Act 1985 prohibits, through criminal sanction, certain activities when carried out on a commercial basis such as advertising for or negotiating surrogacy. The legislation does not outlaw non-profit-making surrogacy agencies. Neither does the Act prohibit the making of surrogacy arrangements, and s.2(2) specifically excludes the surrogate mother and commissioning couple from the provisions of the Act.

Conclusions

Reproductive technology and cloning raise a vast array of novel ethical and legal issues. A great deal of research must have occurred before the birth of the first IVF baby, Louise Brown in 1978. However, there was little public debate on the ethics of reproductive technology at that time.

Assisted reproductive technology accounts for about 1% of live births and raises a variety of novel ethical issues in relation to:
- parenthood
- responsibilities of gamete donors

- anonymity of donors versus rights of offspring to information about their parents
- issues in human embryonic research
- pre-implantation diagnosis
- generation of children for purposes of tissue transplantation
- posthumous conception
- responsibilities and liabilities of healthcare professionals
- legal regulation of reproduction and the role of the HFEA
- the ethical status of the embryo
- patenting of embryonic stem-cell lines.

Many of the issues surround the central issue of the moral status of the human embryo. According to Professor John Wyatt, 'the redefinition of human embryos as mere biological material or "toti-potent stem cells" in order to allay public concerns smacks of semantic trickery rather than responsible debate'.

Those who hold that the human embryo is deserving of respect as a human being will object to both therapeutic and reproductive cloning, irrespective of any potential benefits to others. IVF may be combined with embryo selection prior to implantation, and there is inevitably 'embryo wastage'.

Some would also disallow IVF as the production of a human being within an alien and artificial environment outside the context of normal sexual intercourse. This is giving rise to a new class of litigation brought by the first generations conceived by IVF. They are now of an age to sue in order to discover the identity of their fathers. They may challenge laws that protect the confidentiality of the donor father as being contrary to the human and legal rights of any child so born, including those recognized under Article 8 of the convention.

These 'children of IVF' object to being unable to trace their own genetic ancestry, partly for reasons relating to the health of themselves and their own children (e.g. where there might be a danger of inadvertently marrying within too close degrees of kinship), and partly for psychological and social reasons.

The debate about assisted reproductive techniques throws into the limelight a whole series of issues relating to the status of fathers and the significance of the paternal role in familial relationships and in the upbringing of children. This, in turn, reflects a developing debate about that issue in the wider context of family and medical law. It is likely that these issues will continue to come before the Family Division of the High Court.

Keypoints

- IVF is responsible for a small but significant number of live births.
- Reproductive technology raises a number of complex ethico-legal issues.
- Cloning for reproductive purposes is prohibited by law, while cloning for research ('therapeutic' cloning) is permitted.

Chapter 11

The law in relation to end-of-life issues

Learning objectives

Core knowledge
- Definitions of brain-stem death and PVS
- The law in relation to homicide

Clinical applications
- Withholding and withdrawing treatment in PVS patients
- Organ donation

Background principles and case law
- Physician-assisted suicide and intentional killing
- *Tony Bland* (1993)
- *Diane Pretty* (2002)

Introduction

All clinicians will be involved in the care of dying patients and decisions regarding resuscitation and palliative care. It is important to understand the law in relation to homicide as it is applied to any form of 'medical killing' in the form of physician-assisted suicide or 'mercy killing'. Competent adult patients have a right to accept or refuse life-sustaining treatment. However, decisions have to be made on behalf of premature infants and severely handicapped children by their parents and occasionally by the courts. Decisions may also have to be made regarding the treatment of incapacitated patients who are terminally ill or chronically sick, or who are in the persistent or permanent vegetative state (PVS) or less serious comatose states.

In Scotland, Welfare Attorneys have the power to make decisions on behalf of incapacitated patients. Otherwise it remains the responsibility of doctors, in conjunction with the patient's relatives and other carers, to decide what is in the 'best interests' of the patient.

Definitions

Brain-stem death

In Britain, death is defined clinically as the irreversible destruction of brain-stem function ('brain-stem death'), and can be distinguished from conditions like PVS. Currently there is no statutory definition of death in UK law, although the criteria for brain-stem death have been accepted by the courts throughout the UK and by Coroners. In the rare 'locked-in state' the patient remains conscious but is unable to communicate.

The underlying conditions and diagnostic tests for confirming brain-stem death were defined in the Report of the Conferences of Medical Royal Colleges in 1976 (Table 11.1). The Department of Health issued a Code of Practice for the diagnosis of Brain Stem Death in 1998 that was prepared by the Royal College of Physicians and reiterated the underlying causes of death and diagnostic criteria, while distinguishing death from PVS.

Table 11.1 Diagnosis of brain-stem death

A. Predisposing conditions:

1 The patient should be deeply comatose.

   (a) There should be no suspicion that this state is due to depressant drugs.

   (b) Primary hypothermia as a cause of coma should have been excluded.

   (c) Metabolic and endocrine disturbances that can be responsible for or can contribute to coma should have been excluded.

2 The patient is being maintained on a ventilator because spontaneous respiration had previously become inadequate or had ceased altogether.

3 There should be no doubt that the patient's condition is due to irremediable structural brain damage. The diagnosis of a disorder that can lead to brain-stem death should have been fully established.

B. Diagnostic tests for the confirmation of brain-stem death

'All brain-stem reflexes are absent:

   (i) The pupils are fixed in diameter and do not respond to sharp changes in the intensity of incident light.

   (ii) There is no corneal reflex.

   (iii) The vestibulo-ocular reflexes are absent.

   (iv) No motor response within the cranial nerve distribution can be elicited by adequate stimulation of any somatic area.

   (v) There is no gag reflex response to bronchial stimulation by a suction catheter passed down the trachea.

   (vi) No respiratory movements occur when the patient is disconnected from the mechanical ventilator for long enough to ensure that the arterial carbon dioxide tension rises above the threshold for stimulation of respiration.'

'Diagnosis of Brain Death', *BMJ* 1976;1187.

Additional considerations:

• The diagnostic tests should be repeated at an interval dependent upon the underlying pathology, so as to obviate observer error. The interval between tests might be as long as 24 hours.

• Confirmatory investigations, such as electroencephalography (EEG), cerebral angiography or cerebral blood-flow measurements, are not necessary for the diagnosis. The presence of spinal reflexes does not exclude a diagnosis of brain-stem death.

Table 11.2 Diagnosis of Persistent Vegetative State (PVS)

'A clinical condition of unawareness of self and environment in which the patient breathes spontaneously, has a stable circulation, and shows cycles of eye closure and opening which may simulate sleep and waking. This may be a transient stage in the recovery from coma or it may persist until death.'

J R Coll Physicians Lond. 1996;30:119–21

• The diagnosis ought to be made by an experienced clinician, usually a consultant. A specialist neurologist or neurosurgeon is not normally required except when the primary diagnosis is in doubt.

• The decision to withdraw artificial support should normally be made by a consultant (or his suitably experienced deputy who has been registered for at least 5 years) and one other doctor, once the diagnosis has been made.

Persistent vegetative state

PVS is a rare disorder that is diagnosed on the basis of clinical examination and observation. PVS has been defined by a Working Group of the Royal College of Physicians (Table 11.2).

A diagnosis of a permanent vegetative state may be made when a patient has been in a continuing vegetative state following head injury for more than twelve months or following other causes of brain damage for more than six months.

The cardinal features of PVS are that the patient displays a sleep–wake pattern, responds to stimuli only in a reflex way, and shows no meaningful responses to the environment. The patient may be awake, but lacks awareness.

The diagnosis of PVS is clinical. There are no specific diagnostic tests to diagnose PVS or to predict the potential for recovery. Indeed, the main problem in the diagnosis is the need to prove a negative—the absence of awareness of self and the environment, particularly as it is recognized that (un)awareness is part of a continuum. In the words of the original description of PVS, there must be 'no evidence of a working mind'. The Royal College stresses that the diagnosis is essentially clinical, and must take into account the observations of the carers and family.

A structured systematic approach is recommended to make a diagnosis of PVS, which includes examination for:

- Sustained, reproducible, purposeful or voluntary behavioural responses to noxious visual, auditory, or tactile stimuli.
- Language comprehension or expression.
- Any spontaneous meaningful motor activity (including vocalization).

Patients in PVS may have spontaneous roving eye movements, or look towards the source of a noise or a new visual stimulus, and may even 'track' objects. However, they should not show evidence of responding to direct visual stimuli, as this is considered to require a higher degree of cortical processing. If the patient shows a startle response to a sudden noise, careful observation will be required to determine if the patient can obey simple commands, particularly if the patient is showing signs of spontaneous movement. Indeed some motor activity, e.g. limb movements, grimacing and yawning, is not unusual, both spontaneously and in response to sensory stimuli. Nevertheless, the clinician must determine if there is any co-ordinated movement in relation to nursing manoeuvres or other aspects of care that might signify some residual awareness.

The difficulty in both diagnosing the vegetative state and predicting the outcome of severely brain-damaged patients is illustrated by the finding that of 40 patients referred to the Royal Hospital for Neuro-disability between 1992 and 1995, having been diagnosed as being in a vegetative state by the referring doctor, it was found that only 10 (25%) remained in a persistent or permanent vegetative state, 13 (33%) slowly emerged from the vegetative state during rehabilitation, and 17 (43%) were considered to have been misdiagnosed.

Brain-stem death and organ donation

The law governing cadaveric organ transplantation is the Human Tissue Act 1961, and for dona-

Table 11.3 Human Tissues Act 1961

Under the Act:
- A person may request in writing or orally, in the presence of two witnesses, that his body or any specified part may be used after his death for therapeutic purposes, medical education or research (s.1(1)).
- The person who is 'lawfully in possession' of the body may authorize the removal from the body of 'any part, or, as the case may be, the specified part' to be used in accordance with the request, unless he has reason to believe that a request was subsequently withdrawn (s.1(1)).
- The person 'lawfully in possession of the body' may authorize the removal of any part of the body for therapeutic, education or research purposes (s.1(2)) and may authorize a post mortem examination even if 'not directed or requested by the coroner or any other competent legal authority' (s.2(2)), if having made such 'reasonable enquiry as may be practicable' he has no reason to believe that the deceased person had expressed an objection that has not been withdrawn or that the surviving spouse or any surviving relative of the deceased objects (s.1(2)).

A feature of the Act is the absence of any penalty for non-compliance.

tions from live donors the Human Organ Transplants Act 1989.

The Human Tissue Act 1961 (Table 11.3)

This enables organs and tissues to be used for therapeutic purposes, including transplantation. The Act does not provide a comprehensive regulatory framework. It does not explicitly require consent for the taking, storage or use of organs or tissues. However, 'reasonable enquiry' should be made of relatives to establish a lack of objection where the deceased has not made known his or her wishes. Where a patient dies without expressing their wishes as to whether a post mortem can be carried out and organs can be removed, the Act requires the person 'lawfully in possession of the body' (usually the hospital authorities) to determine whether the 'surviving spouse' or 'any surviving relative' does have any objection. Where the views of the deceased are known, the legal position is clear. However, in practice, doctors tend to respect the views of the relatives if they object to the removal of organs.

The Human Organ Transplants Act 1989

This regulates live organ transplants and commercial dealings for transplantation where organs have been removed from either living or dead people. Under s.1 it is an offence to deal commercially with organs from either living or dead donors where the organs are intended for transplantation.

Euthanasia, assisted suicide and related issues

Deliberate acts of 'mercy killing'

The current state of the law regarding so-called 'mercy killing' was stated by Lord Goff in the case of *Bland v Airedale NHS Trust* (Table 11.4).

Lord Goff said:

'It is not lawful for a doctor to administer a drug to his patient to bring about his death, even though that course is prompted by a humanitarian desire to end his suffering, however great that suffering may be. So to act is to cross the Rubicon which runs between on the one hand the care of the living patient and on the other hand euthanasia—actively causing his death to avoid or end his suffering. Euthanasia is not lawful at common law.'

Lord Goff in *Bland*

Table 11.4 The case of Tony Bland

Tony Bland was a victim of the Hillsborough Football Stadium disaster in 1989. He developed anoxic brain damage as a result of crush injuries and was subsequently diagnosed as having PVS. His doctor and parents had sought declaratory relief from the Court that the deliberate withdrawal so as to end his life of food and fluids administered through a naso-gastric tube would be lawful.

Airedale NHS Trust v Bland (1993)

Furthermore, the consent of the victim would not render 'mercy killing' lawful:

'That "mercy killing" by active means is murder was taken for granted in the directions to the jury in *R v Adams* (Bodkin) (1957), *R v Arthur* (1981) and *R v Cox* (1992) and has never so far as I know been doubted . . . so far as I am aware no satisfactory reason has ever been advanced for suggesting that it makes the least difference in law, as distinct from morals, if the patient consents to or indeed urges the ending of his life by active means.'

Lord Mustill in *Bland*

Omissions that are intended to end life

In the case of *Bland* the issue was whether or not hydration and nutrition, delivered by tube, might be withdrawn from Tony Bland, who suffered from PVS, with the knowledge and intent that this would bring about his death (Table 11.1). Five Law Lords sat on the case.

The life of a patient in PVS may lawfully be terminated by a deliberate omission to provide life-sustaining treatment or sustenance. There remains, in law, a distinction between acts and omissions. As explained by Lord Mustill there is:

'a distinction drawn by the criminal law between acts and omissions, and it carries with it inescapably a distinction between, on the one hand what is often called "mercy-killing", where active steps are taken in a medical context to terminate the life of a suffering patient, and a situation such as the present where the proposed conduct has the aim for equally humane reasons of terminating the life of Anthony Bland by withholding from him the basic necessities of life. The acute unease which I feel about adopting this way through the legal and ethical maze is I believe due in an important part to the sensation that however much the terminologies may differ the ethical status of the two courses of action is for all relevant purposes indistinguishable.'

Lord Mustill in *Bland*

Lord Goff also distinguished between the administering of a lethal drug and the non-provision of treatment:

'The law draws a crucial distinction between cases in which a doctor decides not to provide, or to continue to provide, for his patient treatment or care which could or might prolong his life, and those in which he decides, for example by administering a lethal drug, actively to bring his patient's life to an end. As I have already indicated, the former may be lawful, either because the doctor is giving effect to his patient's wishes by withholding the treatment or care, or even in certain circumstances in which (on principles which I shall describe) the patient is incapacitated from stating whether or not he gives his consent. But it is not lawful for a doctor to administer a drug to his patient to bring about his death, even though that course is prompted by a humanitarian desire to end his suffering, however great that suffering may be':

Lord Goff in *Bland*

The law of murder requires both a guilty intent (*mens rea*) and a guilty act (*actus reus*). In this case it was said that where there is no legal duty of care, there can be no legal *actus reus*, even though the intention of the omission is to bring about the death of the patient. This was an unusual way to put the issue since, under Lord Atkin's neighbour principle in *Donoghue v Stevenson* (1932), everyone has a duty of care not to injure his neighbour by negligence, still less deliberately (albeit by omission). That duty is all the greater, as we have seen, for a doctor having care of a patient. Moreover, in the law of homicide, an omission as well as acts of commission can give rise to criminal liability. It may be for this reason that Lord Mustill later said that the law had been left in a 'misshapen state' after the *Bland* decision.

In the case of Tony Bland it was held that there was no longer a duty of care because of his PVS state—he had no 'best interests', because he had no interests at all. This was graphically stated by Lord Keith:

'It is, however, perhaps permissible to say that to an individual with no cognitive capacity whatever, and no prospect of ever recovering any such capacity in this world, it must be a matter of complete indifference whether he lives or dies.'

Lord Browne-Wilkinson concluded that, while there was the *mens rea* of murder, there was no *actus reus*. Therefore the withdrawal of hydration and nutrition from Tony Bland was not unlawful.

'Murder consists of causing the death of another with intent so to do. What is proposed in the present case is to adopt a course with the intention of bringing about Anthony Bland's death. As to the element of intention or *mens rea*, in my judgment there can be no real doubt that it is present in this case: the whole purpose of stopping artificial feeding is to bring about the death of Anthony Bland. As to the guilty act, or *actus reus*, the criminal law draws a distinction between the commission of a positive act which causes death and the omission to do an act which would have prevented death. In general an omission to prevent death is not an *actus reus* and cannot give rise to a conviction for murder. But where the accused was under a duty to the deceased to do the act which he omitted to do, such omission can constitute the *actus reus* of homicide, either murder (*Rex v. Gibbins* (1918) 13 Cr.App.R. 134) or manslaughter (*Reg. v. Stone* [1977] Q.B. 354) depending upon the *mens rea* of the accused.'

Lord Browne-Wilkinson in *Bland*

Lord Browne-Wilkinson then neatly side-stepped the problem by finding that clinicians had no duty of care to Tony Bland to continue his feeding by tube, and so there was no *actus reus*. In order to achieve this outcome tube-feeding was re-classified as 'treatment' for PVS patients, albeit the actual feeding (which kept Bland alive) was not strictly speaking a form of treatment, since true PVS is permanent and incurable.

This re-definition has not surprisingly resulted in calls for such tube-feeding to be similarly re-classified for other serious comatose conditions. The courts have not been prepared to go that far, although the decision in *Bland* to remove tube-feeding so that death ensued was later held by Dame Elizabeth Butler-Sloss, President of the Family Division of the High Court, to be compatible with Articles 2 and 3 of the European Convention on Human Rights (see *Re: H, Re: M* (2000)).

Practice Note of the Official Solicitor concerning the Vegetative State

Following the Bland judgment, the withdrawal of hydration and nutrition from patients in PVS requires application to the court (Table 11.5).

Physician-assisted suicide

According to Lord Bingham in the case of *R (Pretty) v DPP* (2002):

'The law confers no right to commit suicide. Suicide was always, as a crime, anomalous, since it was the only crime with which no defendant could ever be charged . . . Suicide (and with it attempted suicide) was decriminalized because recognition of the common law offence was not thought to act as a deterrent, because it cast an unwarranted stigma on innocent members of the suicide's family and because it led to the distasteful result that patients recovering in hospital from a failed suicide attempt were prosecuted, in effect, for their lack of success.'

Physician-assisted suicide is undoubtedly unlawful. According to s.2(1) of the Suicide Act 1961:

'2(1)—A person who aids, abets, counsels or procures the suicide of another, or an attempt by another to commit suicide, shall be liable on conviction on indictment to imprisonment for a term not exceeding fourteen years.'

While suicide itself was decriminalized for the victim, aiding or abetting suicide remains an offence, as was explained by Mr Justice Woolf in *A-G v Able* (1984) (the 'EXIT' case):

'S1 of the Act having abrogated the criminal responsibility of the suicide, s.2(1) retains the criminal liability of an accessory at or before the fact. The nature of that liability has, however,

Table 11.5 Practice Note of the Official Solicitor concerning the Vegetative State

In July 1996 the Official Solicitor issued guidance concerning applications to the court before the withdrawal of hydration and nutrition from those with PVS. In summary it said:

1 The termination of artificial feeding and hydration for patients in a vegetative state will in virtually all cases require the prior sanction of a High Court judge.

2 The diagnosis should be made in accordance with the most up-to-date generally accepted guidelines of the medical profession . . . It is not appropriate to apply to court for permission to terminate artificial feeding and hydration until the condition is judged to be permanent. The diagnosis of PVS is not absolute, but based upon probabilities, and should not be made within 12 months of a head injury or within 6 months for other causes of brain damage.

3 Normally the application is for a declaration; but applications to court in relation to minors should be made within wardship. In such cases the applicant should seek the leave of the court for the termination of feeding and hydration, rather than a declaration.

4 The originating summons should be in the following form:
'It is declared that despite the inability of X to give a valid consent, the plaintiffs and/or the responsible medical practitioners
　(i) may lawfully discontinue all life-sustaining treatment and medical support measures (hydration by artificial means) designed to keep X alive in his existing permanent vegetative state; and
　(ii) may lawfully furnish such treatment and nursing care whether at hospital or elsewhere under medical supervision as may be appropriate to ensure X suffers the least distress and retains the greatest dignity until such time as his life comes to an end. . . .

5 The hearing will normally be in open court, with steps taken to preserve the anonymity of the patient and the patient's family. An order restricting publicity will continue to have effect notwithstanding the death of the patient, unless and until an application is made to discharge it.

6 The applicant may be the next of kin or an individual closely connected with the patient or the relevant health authority or NHS trust. Those close to the patient cannot veto an application, but they must be taken fully into account by the court.

7 The Official Solicitor will normally be invited to act as
cont'd

Table 11.5 *Continued*

guardian *ad litem* of the patient, or where he does not represent the patient, he should be joined as a defendant or respondent.

8 There should be at least two independent medical reports on the patient from doctors experienced in assessing disturbances of consciousness.

9 The Official Solicitor's representative will normally be required to interview those close to the patient as well as seeing the patient and those caring for him.

10 The views of the patient may have been previously expressed. The High Court may determine the effect of a purported advance directive as to future medical treatment. The patient's previously expressed views, if any, will be an important component in the decisions of the doctors and of the court, if they are clearly established and intended to apply in the circumstances which have arisen.

Summarized from Practice Note of the Official Solicitor on Vegetative State, July 1996

Table 11.6 The case of Diane Pretty

Mrs Diane Pretty suffered from motor neurone disease and was paralysed from the neck downwards. She wanted to have control over the manner of her death. She was no longer able to commit suicide, and wished her husband to assist her. He agreed. However, the Director of Public Prosecutions (DPP) refused to undertake not to prosecute him for the offence of assisting in her suicide under s.2(1) of the Suicide Act 1961. He therefore sought to challenge the Director's refusal. The case went on appeal to the House of Lords, and eventually was heard in the European Court of Human Rights, which gave judgment shortly before she died in a hospice in England. All judges in all courts unanimously refused to overturn the Director's decision to refuse the advance immunity from prosecution.

R (Pretty) v DPP (2002)

changed. From being a participant in an offence of another, the accessory becomes the principal offender.'

Mr Justice Woolf (now Lord Chief Justice) went on to explain what was the minimum necessary to make a person an accessory before the fact, quoting from *Russell on Crime*:

'. . . the conduct of an alleged accessory should indicate (a) that he knew that the particular deed was contemplated, and (b) that he approved of or assented to it, and (c) that his attitude in respect of it in fact encouraged the principal offender to perform [and I would here add "or to attempt to perform"] the deed.'

Quoting a former Lord Chief Justice, Lord Widgery, from A-G's Reference (1975), he defined procurement as:

'To procure means to produce by endeavour. You procure a thing by setting out to see that it happens and taking the appropriate steps to produce that happening. You cannot procure an offence unless there is a causal link between what you do and the commission of the offence.'

The case of Diane Pretty (Table 11.6)

In the *Pretty* case the House of Lords held that the Convention did not oblige a state to legalize assisted suicide.

Article 2:

• did not acknowledge that it was for the individual to choose whether to live or die, nor did it protect a right of self-determination in relation to issues of life and death; and

• enunciated the principle of the sanctity of life and provided a guarantee that no individual should be deprived of life by means of intentional human intervention, but did not provide or protect a 'right to die'.

The European Court of Human Rights held:

• the convention did not guarantee a right to assisted suicide;

• no right to die could be derived from the right to life;

• there was no ill-treatment by the Government, and the medical authorities were providing adequate care;

• there was no breach of the prohibition of inhumane or degrading treatment (Article 3);

• the blanket ban on assisted suicide under the Suicide Act 1961 was not disproportionate.

Table 11.7 The case of Ms B

Miss B, a 43-year-old former social worker, suffered a bleed from a spinal haemangioma. She was admitted to hospital in 1999 for about 5 weeks, and her condition improved. She recovered to the extent that she was able to go back to work. However, at the beginning of 2001 she had a further bleed that caused severe cord damage, and she became tetraplegic. She was placed on a ventilator, upon which she was entirely dependent for survival. She subsequently asked for the ventilation to be discontinued. Dame Elizabeth Butler-Sloss, President of the Family Division of the High Court, ruled that she had the 'necessary mental capacity to give consent or to refuse consent to life-sustaining medical treatment'. She held that Miss B could be transferred to another hospital and the ventilator could be withdrawn in accordance with her wishes, with any treatment necessary to 'ease her suffering and permit her life to end peacefully and with dignity'.

She died on 29 April 2002 after ventilation was withdrawn.

B v An NHS Trust (2002)

The case of Ms B (2002)

In contrast to Diane Pretty, who wanted the assistance of her husband actively to bring about her death, Ms B was on a ventilator and wished it to be withdrawn as treatment (Table 11.7).

A crucial question was posed by her counsel, Mr Francis QC, who asked whether it was her wish to die, or not to remain alive in the present condition, to which she replied: 'The latter . . . given the range of choices, I would want to recover and have my life back, or significant enough recovery to have a better quality of life. I am not convinced from the evidence that that is going to happen, and I find the idea of living like this intolerable.'

Hence there was a significant difference between wishing positively to end a life (in effect a suicidal wish) and not wanting to continue living attached to a ventilator (in effect a legitimate refusal of treatment by a competent patient). It was decided that she was mentally capable of making a decision regarding the withdrawal of ventilation. As it was her clear wish to discontinue ventilation, this wish was granted by the court in accordance with established legal principle.

Cases

A number of doctors have been on trial before the courts or the GMC for helping patients to die. Their cases are illustrative.

Dr John Bodkin Adams (1957)

Dr John Bodkin Adams was an Eastbourne GP who was charged with the murder of an elderly patient. He was accused of administering pain-relieving drugs in order to cause her death. During the trial at the Old Bailey, it was alleged that he had benefited from her will to the tune of £157,000. He was acquitted. The case is important for a recognition by Mr Justice Devlin (later Lord Devlin) of the principle of double or dual effect, when he held that:

'. . . a doctor is entitled to do all that is proper and necessary to relieve pain even if the measure he took might incidentally shorten life by hours or perhaps longer'.

Dr Leonard Arthur 1981

Dr Leonard Arthur stood trial at Leicester Crown Court for the attempted murder of John Pearson, a newborn baby with Down's syndrome. His mother had rejected him, and Dr Arthur, a highly respected paediatrician, had written in the notes after seeing both parents: 'Parents do not wish the baby to survive. Nursing care only.'

Baby Pearson was then given dihydrocodeine (DF118) 'as required' in dosages of up to 5 mg at four-hourly intervals (the firm manufacturing the drug does not recommend that it be given to any baby under 4 years old). John died about 54 hours after birth. The stated cause of death was bronchopneumonia as a result of Down's syndrome.

There was doubt as to the cause of death, and Mr Justice Farquharson directed that the charge should be one of attempted murder. The judge said that the distinction between acts and omissions was crucial, and that it was for the jury to say whether '. . . there was an act properly so called on the part of Dr Arthur, as distinct from simply allowing the child to die'.

He also stated that: 'However serious the case may be, however much the disadvantage of being a mongol, indeed, any other handicapped child, no doctor has the right to kill it.'

In accordance with the *Bodkin Adams* case, the judge stated that the administration of a drug by a doctor when it is necessary to relieve pain is a proper medical practice even when the doctor knows that the drugs will themselves cause the patient's death, provided the death is not intended. Therefore, if the purpose of giving DF118 was to prevent suffering, it might be justified on this principle. However, there was some evidence that the effect of the drug would be to stop the child seeking sustenance—something that Dr Arthur had admitted to the police. In the event Dr Arthur was acquitted.

Dr Nigel Cox (1992)

Dr Nigel Cox, a consultant rheumatologist, was charged with, and found guilty of, the attempted murder of 70-year-old Mrs Lillian Boyes. She was a long-standing patient of Dr Cox with intractable pain due to vertebral fractures, leg ulcers and severe rheumatoid arthritis. Dr Cox gave her an injection of potassium chloride. The charges were brought after cremation of the body, and it was never possible to prove that the injection had caused the death. The 12 months' sentence was suspended, and the GMC subsequently allowed Dr Cox to continue to practise medicine after a reprimand.

Dr Nigel Cox remains the only doctor ever to be convicted in the UK of attempting to perform a so-called 'mercy killing'.

Dr Ken Taylor (1995)

Mrs Ormerod, who was 85 years old, had suffered from a series of strokes, senile dementia and mild Parkinson's disease. She was bed-bound. Her GP, Dr Ken Taylor, had taken a decision to withhold nutritional supplements from her, and she died weighing less than 4 stone two months later, although she had been fed by the nurses at the home contrary to the doctor's orders. Dr Taylor was found

guilty of serious professional misconduct by the GMC, and suspended from the medical register for six months. He had failed to perform an adequate assessment of the patient and to take into consideration the views of others involved in the patient's care. He also should have recognized the limits of his professional competence and should have sought a second opinion.

Dr David Moor (1999)

A Newcastle GP, Dr Moor, was accused of giving a lethal dose of diamorphine to an 85-year-old patient, Mr George Liddell, who was thought to be in the terminal stages of bowel cancer. The stated purpose of the injection was to ensure that Mr Liddell had no breakthrough pain. What was unusual in this case was that Dr Moor had told a journalist that he had agreed with the views of Dr Michael Irwin in an article in *The Sunday Times* that had appeared only the day after Mr Liddell's death, in which Dr Irwin had admitted to participating in physician-assisted suicide. Dr Moor said that he had given many of his patients diamorphine to help them have a pain-free death. 'Basically, you address their problems and address their needs and if they have a lot of pain, if they have a lot of suffering, and if the patient's relatives are suffering then you address that with care, compassion and consideration—I would certainly say that over the years I have helped a lot of people to die.' However, although he admitted that he had given Mr Liddell diamorphine to relieve pain, he said that he had not deliberately set out to kill him.

Dr Moor had retired by the time of his trial, and died in 2000.

Dr Harold Shipman (2000)

Dr Harold Shipman was convicted in 2000 of murdering 15 elderly patients and sentenced to prison for life. The later investigation said Shipman had murdered at least 200 other people since 1975, and raised questions about how he was able to evade detection for so many years. High Court Judge Janet Smith, who investigated Shipman's activities after he was jailed, concluded in 2002 that he had killed 215 of his patients, including 171 women and 44 men.

Judge Smith said that she also found a 'real suspicion' that Shipman was responsible for 45 other deaths, and that there was insufficient evidence to form any conclusion in another 38 deaths.

Dr Shipman was later found to have hanged himself in Wakefield Prison in June 2003.

Conclusion

Lord Mustill in *Bland* expressed the view that it was for Parliament to consider the ethical, legal and social issues surrounding cases such as *Bland*. The House of Lords Select Committee in 1993 opposed legalizing euthanasia and assisted suicide. English law now accepts that the lives of those in PVS can be terminated by omission of assisted hydration with the sanction of the courts. 'Mercy killing' remains illegal, together with assisted suicide, and both the English Courts and the European Court of Human Rights have ruled that there is no 'right to die' under Article 2 of the Convention of Human Rights.

Keypoints

- Brain-stem death is regarded as death in the UK.
- The courts have sanctioned the withdrawal of hydration and nutrition for patients with PVS.
- 'Mercy killing' remains unlawful.
- The European Court of Human Rights in Strasbourg has not sanctioned a right to assisted suicide.

Chapter 12

The ethics of end-of-life issues

Physician-assisted suicide and euthanasia

'I will give no deadly drug to anyone, though it be asked of me, nor will I counsel such.'

Hippocratic Oath

'Euthanasia is a deliberate act or omission whose primary intention is to end another's life.'

BMA Medical Ethics Department. Physician Assisted Suicide Project. March 2000.

Crossing the Rubicon. Causing death through deliberate acts or omissions

The landmark case of *Bland* (1993) raised the issue of whether or not hydration and nutrition, deliv-

ered by tube, might be withdrawn knowing and intending that this would bring about his death. One Law Lord said:

'The proposed conduct has the aim . . . of terminating the life of Anthony Bland: the conduct . . . is intended to be the cause of death.'

Lord Mustill in *Bland*

Others said:

'The whole purpose of stopping artificial feeding is to bring about the death of Anthony Bland.'

Lord Browne-Wilkinson in *Bland*

'The intention to bring about the patient's death is there.'

Lord Lowry in *Bland*

However, Lord Goff continued to draw the traditional legal distinction between causing death through acts and by omission, as we saw in the last chapter.

The ethical basis of the decision in Bland has been challenged, not least by the Lords themselves. Lord Mustill expressed 'acute unease' in 'adopting this way through the legal and ethical maze'. In dismissing the appeal (and bringing about the death of Tony Bland) he said

'I fear that your Lordships' House may only emphasise the distortions of a legal structure which is already both morally and intellectually misshapen.'

Lord Browne-Wilkinson commented that:

'the conclusion I have reached will appear to some to be almost irrational. How can it be lawful to allow a patient to die slowly, though painlessly, over a period of weeks from lack of food but unlawful to produce his immediate death by a lethal injection, thereby saving his family from yet another ordeal to add to the tragedy that has already struck them? I find it difficult to find a moral answer to that question.'

Lord Goff asked:

'Why is it that the doctor who gives his patient a lethal injection which kills him commits an unlawful act and indeed is guilty of murder, whereas a doctor who, by discontinuing life support, allows his patient to die, may not act unlawfully and will not do so, if he commits no breach of duty to his patient?'

As Lord Browne-Wilkinson held, there was no doubt that there was the intention, i.e. *mens rea* (guilty intent), to bring about death by not feeding the patient, as we see from the quotation above.

The House of Lords has recognized that, in the case of PVS patients, death may lawfully be brought about through the withdrawal of hydration and nutrition. While their Lordships decided the case as a matter of law, it is still much puzzled over as a matter of medical ethics. To adopt a course of action with the intention of deliberately bringing about the death of a patient seems to be a significant departure from the Hippocratic tradition of medicine.

Physician-assisted suicide and voluntary euthanasia

The House of Lords Select Committee on Medical Ethics in 1994 recommended no change in the law regarding either assisted suicide or voluntary euthanasia. The government has said that it has no plans to depart from this recommendation.

Assisted suicide

The House of Lords Select Committee said this:

'As far as assisted suicide is concerned, we see no reason to recommend any change in the law. We identify no circumstances in which assisted suicide should be permitted, nor do we see any reason to distinguish between the act of a doctor or of any other person in this connection.'

Voluntary euthanasia

On voluntary euthanasia it had this to say:

'The right to refuse medical treatment is far removed from the right to request assistance in dying.

We do not believe that these arguments are sufficient reason to weaken society's prohibition of intentional killing. That prohibition is the cornerstone of law and of social relationships. It protects each one of us impartially, embodying the belief that all are equal. The death of a person affects the lives of others, often in ways and to an extent which cannot be foreseen. We believe that the issue of euthanasia is one in which the interest of the individual cannot be separated from the interest of society as a whole.

To distinguish between murder and "mercy killing" would be to cross the line which prohibits intentional killing, a line which we think it essential to preserve.'

House of Lords Select Committee on Medical Ethics. 1994.

A very similar stance was taken by the Council of Europe's Recommendation 1418 (1999) regarding the protection of the human rights and dignity of the terminally ill and dying. (Table 12.1).

Decisions to withhold or withdraw life-sustaining treatment

Is there a distinction between treatment and care?

In the *Bland* judgment tube feeding was, for the first time, regarded as 'medical treatment', at least for patients in Permanent or Persistent Vegetative State (PVS), and as such could legally be denied to a patient. However, historically both the law and

Table 12.1 Council of Europe: the protection of the human rights and dignity of the terminally ill and dying

The Assembly therefore recommends that the Committee of Ministers encourage the member states of the Council of Europe to respect and protect the dignity of terminally ill or dying persons in all respects . . . by upholding the prohibition against intentionally taking the life of terminally ill or dying persons, while:
(i) recognizing that the right to life, especially with regard to a terminally ill or dying person, is guaranteed by the member states, in accordance with Article 2 of the European Convention on Human Rights, which states that 'no one shall be deprived of his life intentionally';
(ii) recognizing that a terminally ill or dying person's wish to die never constitutes any legal claim to die at the hand of another person;
(iii) recognizing that a terminally ill or dying person's wish to die cannot of itself constitute a legal justification to carry out actions intended to bring about death.

Council of Europe's Recommendation 1418 (1999)

medicine have regarded hydration and nutrition as care rather than as 'medical treatment'.

Medical treatment is disease-specific. The purpose of medical treatment is to prevent or treat disease and to alleviate pain and distress, particularly when cure is not possible. Care refers to those things that are necessary in both health and disease to sustain life. Thus the provision of hydration and nutrition, warmth, shelter, comfort and companionship is ordinarily care, not treatment. Nutrition and hydration serve physiological functions required to sustain life. Hunger and thirst are not diseases to be 'treated' by feeding, but a requirement for the sustenance of all human life. Even for a patient suffering from an eating disorder like anorexia nervosa, where food has a treatment aspect, it nevertheless still remains a requirement for the sustenance of life. Conversely, if nutrition and hydration are treatment, what diseases do they treat or cure? Tube feeding was regarded as treatment for PVS in the case of *Bland*. However, PVS is by definition incurable. It is therefore difficult to see how nutrition and hydration could be said to be 'treatment' for the condition.

Ordinarily there is a presumption in favour of providing food and fluids and ordinary medical treatment to a non-dying patient by whatever means are appropriate for that patient in their particular circumstances. Indeed, the provision of food and fluids is a human right under Articles 2 and 3 of the Convention, given that without food and fluid a patient will inevitably die of hunger and thirst.

However, in the case of *Re: H, Re: M* (2000) the President of the Family Division, Dame Elizabeth Butler-Sloss, found that the removal of tube feeding from two patients in PVS or near-PVS did not breach their human rights. The court reasoned that if the tube-feeding was treatment, then it could be withdrawn if the doctor, in his professional judgement, believed it was not in the patient's best interests and his view passed the *Bolam* test (i.e. a group of doctors expert in that area of practice would have done the same). In this the President adopted the reasoning of Lord Browne-Wilkinson in *Bland*. However, the *Bolam* test being a test for clinical negligence, it was not entirely clear how it applied to a case where:
1 the doctor was considering non-clinical 'best interests' (for which clinical competence is not relevant); and
2 the intention in withdrawing the treatment was to bring about a homicide, which is ordinarily a trespass to the person and not merely negligence, and thus not an issue to which the *Bolam* test would normally apply.
Moreover, the President found that 'deprivation of life' had to import a positive act that was absent here. But it was not clear how a removal of sustenance with the intention of ending a life was not a positive act to deprive the person of life. Moreover, there is a positive duty on the state under Article 2 to take steps to protect life, as the court emphasized in the Gibraltar 'Death on the rock' case (*McCann v UK* (1995)) and in *Osman v UK* (1999), both cases cited to the court. In *Osman* the European Court held that the authorities must do:

'all that could be reasonably expected of them to avoid a real and immediate risk to life of which they have or ought to have knowledge'.

It was not clear how stopping a patient's food and fluids (however delivered) was something less than a 'real and immediate risk to life' that the authorities knew about.

Thus the re-classification of tube feeding as no more than 'treatment' for a PVS patient has had wide-reaching legal, ethical and medical consequences.

Since this case was a decision at High Court level, it may well be re-visited at a higher level in the future, and these issues may be clarified further.

Proportionate and disproportionate means of treatment

Traditionally a distinction has been made in medical ethics between proportionate and disproportionate treatment (this has sometimes been referred to as ordinary and extraordinary treatment). Proportionate treatment means treatment where:

- there is hope of benefit to the patient, i.e. it is not futile;
- the treatment is in 'common use', i.e. it is not experimental;
- it is proportionate to the patient's needs and circumstances;
- it does not pose an undue risk;
- it is not unduly burdensome to the patient;
- and it is not otherwise unreasonable.

Disproportionate means have been regarded as 'over-zealous' treatment in relation to the expected benefits for the patient. While proportionate forms of treatment should be recommended by doctors, neither patients nor doctors should feel obliged to pursue 'over-zealous' or disproportionate therapy.

The distinction between proportionate and disproportionate means is an attempt to provide an ethical framework for guiding clinical decision-making. It focuses upon the physician's perspective of the treatment needs of the individual patient, rather than the disease and its therapy seen in isolation. The proportionate/ disproportionate distinction should be seen in terms of the treatment of a particular patient in their individual circumstances. It is the patient who is being treated, not merely the disease alone.

Clinical decision-making is a continuous interactive process between doctor and patient. The clinician seeks to determine what is in the patient's best clinical interests by the application of his professional skill and judgement.

The clinician then presents the patient with the treatment options and an assessment of the risks, benefits and alternatives.

The patient will then normally consent or refuse according to his assessment of his own overall best interests. The patient may bring a range of non-clinical considerations to his decision, because it is his person and life that will be affected.

What is proportionate for one patient may be disproportionate for another. Moreover, a treatment that is disproportionate in a strictly clinical sense might not be so overall, as a result of some pressing extra-clinical factors. An example might be a man with alcoholic liver disease who has a wife with severe multiple sclerosis and two small children. He may be more willing to abstain totally from alcohol and undergo transplantation because of the needs of his wife and family, who are dependent upon him.

His death from untreated liver disease would so adversely affect his wife and children that the transplant becomes a proportionate treatment in his case, taking into account all the circumstances. In this case the patient's desire to help his family improves his motivation to abstain and to undergo the rigours of the operation. This in turn has a further clinical resonance, since strong motivation may influence the successful outcome of the procedure. Thus do clinical and extra-clinical criteria coalesce.

The point to be made here is that proportionality can only be assessed in the light of each individual patient's circumstances. It is, after all, the patient who will experience the potential benefit or harm of the treatment, and there may be other factors that the clinician has to consider in meeting the patient's overall needs.

Withholding and withdrawing treatment

The withdrawal of treatment should not be made

with the intention of causing harm to the patient, much less to bring about the patient's death. In his oral evidence to the Joint Committee on the Draft Mental Incapacity Bill, Dr Wilks, Chairman of the BMA Medical Ethics Committee, pointed out that:

'Any doctor who makes a decision that someone's life in common parlance has no value and should be terminated and ends treatment with the intention of terminating life is acting illegally and unethically.'

Dr Michael Wilks. 8 October 2003

Hence the central ethical issue is the value of the treatment to the patient rather than the value of the patient's life.

GMC Guidance: Withholding and Withdrawing Life-prolonging Treatments: Good Practice in Decision-making (August 2002)

In the case of patients who are in the process of dying, the GMC points out that the provision of hydration and nutrition may not always be appropriate. The main issue for the dying patient is the relief of distressing symptoms of thirst.

'Where death is imminent, in judging the benefits, burdens or risks, it usually would not be appropriate to start either artificial hydration or nutrition, although artificial hydration provided by the less invasive measures may be appropriate where it is considered that this would be likely to provide symptom relief.'

'Where death is not imminent, it usually will be appropriate to provide artificial nutrition or hydration . . . However, circumstances may arise where you judge that a patient's condition is so severe, and the prognosis so poor, that providing artificial nutrition or hydration may cause suffering, or be too burdensome in relation to the possible benefits.'

However, it will rarely, if ever, be the case that hydration and nutrition are withdrawn from the non-dying patient (who is not in PVS), knowing that the patient will die as a consequence. Nevertheless the GMC mentions that circumstances could arise where the provision of hydration and nutrition might be too burdensome in relation to the possible benefits to the patient.

There will be few circumstances in practice where it is not possible to provide hydration and nutrition to patients who are not in the process of dying. We can think of only two.

• Where there is an intact gastro-intestinal tract and long-term enteral nutrition is required, but it is not feasible to place a gastrosotomy feeding (PEG) tube without serious risk. Such a situation might arise where it is necessary to place the PEG under general anaesthetic, but the risks of anaesthesia are considered unacceptable.

• Where the patient does not have an intact gastro-intestinal tract and requires long-term total parenteral nutrition (TPN) through a central venous line.

However, in both the above circumstances failure to institute long-term feeding by PEG or TPN could not be construed as a deliberate intention to stop feeding the patient. Nevertheless, they might fulfil the conditions specified by the GMC above for not providing 'artificial' hydration and nutrition.

At the time of writing the GMC guidelines are being challenged in the High Court by Mr Leslie Burke, who is a patient with cerebellar ataxia. Mr Burke does not want doctors to decide to withdraw food and fluids or treatment with the intention of ending his life in the event of his becoming incapacitated. He claims that the GMC guidance quoted above is not sufficiently clear and unambiguous so as to remain within the law.

Conscientious objection to withholding or withdrawing treatment

The GMC recognizes that the withdrawal or withholding of life-sustaining treatment may cause difficulty for some doctors, and therefore it makes provision for conscientious objection.

'Where a decision to withhold or withdraw life-prolonging treatment has been made by a competent adult patient, or made by the senior clinician responsible for the care of a patient who lacks capacity to decide (following discussions with those close to the patient and the health care team) doctors who have a conscientious objection to the decision may withdraw from the care of that patient.'

Palliative care

The hospice movement has had a tremendous effect on the management of the terminally ill, not only within the hospices themselves but also outside the movement. Good palliative medicine already enjoys widespread public support.

Palliative care is aimed at the prevention or the alleviation of distressing symptoms, especially in the dying patient. Where a patient is deemed to be dying, it may well be appropriate to withdraw treatment. This means the withholding of 'overzealous' treatment and not the deliberate intent to cause the patient's death. There is an important distinction to be made between the mere foreseeability of death and the intention to cause death. There is also the question of the cause of death. A doctor is not necessarily culpable because the patient died of terminal malignancy. However, it is a different matter if it is intended to bring about the death of a patient who was not otherwise dying. That is currently illegal, and may be a culpable homicide unless the patient is in PVS or near-PVS and a court order has been obtained to withdraw tube feeding.

Hence, the distinction made by the National Council for Hospice and Specialist Palliative Care Services:

'A decision to forgo extraordinary means rests on a recognition that the means of preserving life or restoring health are being forgone because they are no longer beneficial, are no longer useful or are too burdensome. It is not a decision that the life of the patient is no longer one worthy of being lived.'

Ethics Working Party July 1997.

Principle of Double or Dual Effect (Table 12.2)

The Principle of Double or Dual Effect applies where the primary end of a particular procedure or

Table 12.2 Principle of Double or Dual Effect

An action (e.g. an operation or a medical treatment) is morally justified, even when it has harmful side-effects, if:
1. The action itself is ethically good, or at least ethically neutral.
2. The harmful effects are not deliberately intended.
3. The beneficial effects arise from the action itself and not from the harmful effects.
4. There is a sufficient margin of good over harmful effects of the action.

treatment is good and there is a sufficient balance of good over potential harmful effects. The primary end is intended by the operator; the side-effects are not.

The principle was adumbrated by Mr Justice Devlin in the case of *R v Bodkin Adams* (1957) (referred to in Chapter 11) in relation to the use of pain-killing drugs that may have the unintended side-effect of shortening life. Interestingly, however, the proper use of opiate analgesics is now more likely to prolong, rather than shorten, life. Nevertheless, whilst the dangers of opiates may have been overstressed in the past in this context, the principle still applies to many other aspects of medical practice outside palliative care.

In *Bodkin Adams* Mr Justice Devlin (later Lord Devlin) said:

'If the purpose of medicine, the restoration of health, can no longer be achieved there is still much for a doctor to do, and he is entitled to do all that is proper and necessary to relieve pain and suffering, even if the measures he takes may incidentally shorten life... "Cause" means nothing philosophical or technical or scientific. It means what you twelve men and women sitting as a jury in the jury box would regard in a common-sense way as the cause... But, it remains the fact, and it remains the law, that no doctor, nor any man, no more in the case of the dying man than of the healthy, has the right deliberately to cut the thread of life.'

Mr Justice Devlin in *R v Bodkin Adams* (1957)

Table 12.3 The Principle of Double Effect in relation to the use of pain-killing drugs

Double Effect
'243. Some witnesses suggested that the double effect of some therapeutic drugs when given in large doses was being used as a cloak for what in effect amounted to widespread euthanasia, and suggested that this implied medical hypocrisy. We reject that charge while acknowledging that the doctor's intention, and evaluation of the pain and distress suffered by the patient, are of critical significance in judging double effect. If this intention is the relief of severe pain or distress, and the treatment given is appropriate to that end, then the possible double effect should be no obstacle to such treatment being given. Some may say that the intention is not readily ascertainable. But juries are asked every day to assess intention in all sorts of cases, and could do so in respect of double effect if in a particular instance there was any reason to suspect that the doctor's primary intention was to kill the patient rather than to relieve pain and suffering.
244. A doctor called to testify in the case of Dr Bodkin Adams asserted that a particular dose must certainly kill, only to be told that the patient had previously been given that dose and had survived. The primary effect (relief of pain and distress) can be predicted with reasonable confidence but there can be no certainty that the secondary effect (shortening of life) will result. Decisions about dosage are not easy, but the practice of medicine is all about the weighing of risks and benefits.'
The House of Lords Select Committee on Medical Ethics, 1994

In 1960 Lord Devlin observed in a lecture that:

'The law might regard negligent treatment as a new and supervening cause of death, but proper medical treatment consequent upon illness or injury plays no part in legal causation; and to relieve the pains of death is undoubtedly proper medical treatment.'

The House of Lords Select Committee on Medical Ethics reinforced Mr Justice Devlin's view of Double Effect (Table 12.3).

Decisions relating to Cardiopulmonary Resuscitation (CPR)

Introduction

A joint statement was recently issued by the British Medical Association, the Resuscitation Council (UK) and the Royal College of Nursing regarding Cardiopulmonary Resuscitation (CPR) and Do Not Resuscitate (DNR) orders called *Decisions Relating to Cardiopulmonary Resuscitation, 2001*.

Summary of recommendations

The following is a summary of the main recommendations of the Guidelines issued in the joint statement ('the Guidelines').

Principles

- Information about CPR and the chances of success must be realistic.
- Sensitive discussion should be encouraged, but not forced.
- Decisions should be based on the needs of individual patients and reviewed regularly.
- Timely support for patients and those close to them and effective sensitive communication is essential.

Practical issues

- Information concerning CPR should be available to patients and staff.
- Leaflets should be available to patients, and those close to them, explaining how decisions concerning CPR are made.
- Decisions regarding CPR should be effectively communicated to healthcare professionals.

In Emergencies where no decision has been made about CPR

CPR should be attempted unless:
- the patient has refused CPR;

- the patient is clearly in a terminal phase of illness; or
- the burdens of the treatment outweigh the benefits.

Advance Decision-Making

- Competent patients should be involved in decision-making unless they indicate they do not wish to be.
- In the case of incompetent patients, people close to them can be helpful in reflecting their views.

Clinical Guidelines

Hospitals, general practices, residential care homes and ambulance services are now required to have policies regarding CPR that respect patients' rights and are accessible to the relevant staff.

Death is inevitable for all, and CPR could theoretically be applied to everyone prior to death. However, it is clearly important to identify those patients in whom death is imminent or inevitable, for whom cardiopulmonary arrest would be a terminal event, and where CPR would be inappropriate.

While there is a general presumption in favour of CPR, it 'is unlikely to be considered reasonable to attempt to resuscitate a patient who is in the terminal phase of illness or for whom the burdens of the treatment clearly outweigh the potential benefits'.

According to the Guidelines:

'Decisions about whether to attempt to resuscitate a particular patient are made in advance as part of overall care planning for that patient and, as such, are discussed with the patient along with other aspects of future care.'

A decision not to resuscitate should only be made after appropriate consultation and consideration of all the relevant aspects of the patient's condition, including:

- the likely clinical outcome, including the likelihood of successfully restarting the patient's heart and breathing, and the overall benefit achieved from a successful resuscitation;
- the patient's known, or ascertainable wishes;

- the patient's human rights, including the right to life and the right to be free from degrading treatment; and
- the views of all members of the medical and nursing team, including those involved in the patient's primary and secondary care and, with due regard to patient confidentiality, the people close to the patient.

Specific issues relating to competent patients

The need to discuss CPR

Patients have an ethical and legal right to information regarding their health and decisions relating to them. Discussions regarding CPR are sensitive and often complex, and should be undertaken by senior members of the medical and nursing teams. The Guidelines recommend that information about resuscitation should be included in the general literature provided to patients and should be readily available to all patients and to people close to the patient. Where patients are 'at risk' of arrest or have terminal illness, discussions should still occur regarding CPR, unless the patient indicates unwillingness to discuss this issue.

'Where competent patients are at foreseeable risk of cardiopulmonary arrest, or have terminal illness, there should be sensitive exploration of their wishes regarding resuscitation. This will normally arise as part of general discussions about that patient's care. Information should not be forced on unwilling recipients, however, and if patients indicate that they do not wish to discuss resuscitation this should be respected.'

Decisions Relating to Cardiopulmonary Resuscitation, 2001.

Patient requests for CPR where resuscitation is deemed clinically inappropriate

The best chances of a successful outcome from CPR are when defibrillators are readily available, e.g. in Casualty, ITU or CCU and in patients suffering from VF arrest who do not have significant co-morbidity. For many patients a decision not to re-suscitate is made when resuscitation is unlikely to be successful or it is considered futile because the patient is in the final stages of a terminal illness. The guidance points out that 'doctors cannot be required to give treatment contrary to their clinical judgment, but should, whenever possible, respect patients' wishes to receive treatment which carries only a very small chance of success or benefit'.

Incapacitated adults

In England and Wales, no one, other than a doctor or the court, is entitled to make clinical decisions on behalf of a mentally incapacitated adult.

- Those close to the patient should be kept informed about the patient's health and be involved in decision-making in order to reflect the patient's view and preferences.
- It should be made clear that their role is not to take decisions on behalf of the patient (this is not the case in Scotland).
- While it is good practice to involve those close to the patient, the guidance rightly points out that 'the information sought from people close to patients is to help ascertain what the patient would have wanted in these circumstances, as opposed to what those consulted would like for the patient or what they would want for themselves if they were in the same situation'.

However, in Scotland, the Adults with Incapacity (Scotland) Act 2000 allows those over 16 years to appoint a proxy decision-maker who has the legal power to make decisions when the patient loses capacity. Nevertheless, according to the Guidelines :

'proxy decision makers cannot demand treatment which is judged to be contrary to the patient's interests. The Act also requires doctors to take account, so far as is reasonable and practicable, of the views of the patient's nearest relative and his or her primary carer.'

Decisions Relating to Cardiopulmonary Resuscitation, 2001.

Children and young people

Medical decisions regarding children and young people should normally be made in conjunction with parents. Young patients below the age of 16 who are 'Gillick competent' can give consent to medical treatment, but their refusal can be overridden by the parents. However:

'where a competent young person refuses treatment, the harm caused by violating the young person's choice must be balanced against the harm caused by failing to treat.'

Decisions Relating to Cardiopulmonary Resuscitation, 2001.

The European Court of Human Rights has taken the view that parents do have the right under Article 8 of the European Convention to be involved in decision-making on behalf of their children.

W v UK (1987) involved the right of parents to be involved in decisions concerning children taken into care. The European Court asked whether, having regard to the particular circumstances of the case and notably the serious nature of the decisions to be taken, the parents have been involved in the decision-making process to a degree sufficient to provide them with the requisite protection of their interests.

However, in March 2004, the European Court decided unanimously in the case of David Glass (*Glass v. the United Kingdom*, application no. 61827/00) that the administration of diamorphine to David by doctors at St Mary's Hospital, Portsmouth, in the face of parental opposition was a breach of the boy's rights under Article 8 by reason of an unwarranted invasion of his physical integrity and private life. Relatives had tried to prevent the administration of diamorphine by physical restraint, and had later been convicted by a criminal court for assault.

Do Not Resuscitate (DNR) Orders

The Guidelines consider three circumstances when resuscitation would be inappropriate.

1 'Where attempting CPR will not start the patient's heart and breathing.'

This can be justified on the basis of futility.

2 'Where there is no benefit in restarting the patient's heart and breathing.'

The circumstances envisaged here are where CPR will only gain a very brief extension of life, because imminent death cannot be averted, and where the patient will never have awareness or the ability to interact, and therefore cannot experience benefit.

3 'Where the expected benefit is outweighed by the burdens.'

CPR carries a risk of significant side-effects such as sternal or rib fractures, splenic rupture and anoxic brain damage. CPR may also be traumatic for a conscious patient and the relatives.

The courts have confirmed that it is lawful to withhold CPR where it is felt it would not confer a benefit on the patient in terms of the likely outcome and quality of life for the patient.

The case of *Re R (adult: medical treatment)* (1996)

This is an important case in which the court was asked to decide the place of DNRs (Table 12.4).

The courts are reluctant to substitute judicial for clinical judgement. Sir Stephen Brown endorsed the guidelines produced by the relevant professional organizations—in this case the 1993 guidelines of the BMA and RCN. He said:

'These guidelines, therefore, should be viewed as a framework, providing basic principles within which decisions regarding local policies on CPR may be formulated. Further assistance for doctors and nurses, where individual problems arise, can be obtained from their respective professional organizations.'

The issue of withdrawing hydration and nutrition was not considered since, at the time of the hearing, it had been decided to insert a gastrostomy feeding tube.

Sir Stephen Brown stressed that the management of R did not include any action that would be aimed at causing his death, and that his treatment should rest with those with clinical responsibility in conjunction with his parents.

Table 12.4 The case of *Re R (adult: medical treatment)* (1996)

R was a 23-year-old man with cerebral palsy. The evidence was that:

'He is not in the category of someone in the persistent vegetative state, but in the scale of gravity of the low awareness state he would rate between 1 and 2 on the scale of 10. He appears to respond to pain, and grimaces, but Dr Andrews is not sure whether he really feels it. He is totally dependent.'

Dr S, a consultant with a special interest in learning disabilities, felt that R's condition was 'deteriorating neurologically and physically' as he weighed only 5 stone and had recurrent chest infections, severe constipation, bleeding from an ulcerated oesophagus, epileptic fits, dehydration and under-nutrition. Dr S signed a 'do not resuscitate order' with the agreement of the parents. However, certain members of staff became concerned, and the NHS Trust applied to the Family Division of the High Court for declaratory relief that, in the event of R requiring CPR, or treatment of a life-threatening condition, it would be lawful for his doctors:

1) to withhold such life-sustaining treatment and medical support measures designed to keep the defendant alive in his existing catastrophically brain-damaged state, including:
   (i) resuscitation and ventilation;
   (ii) nutrition and hydration by artificial means;
   (iii) the administration of antibiotics;
2) to furnish such treatment and nursing care as may be appropriate to ensure that R suffers the least distress and retains the greatest dignity until such time as his life comes to an end.

'In this case there is no question of the court being asked to approve a course aimed at terminating his life or accelerating death. The court is concerned with circumstances in which steps should not be taken to prolong his death.'

He declared that, although R could not himself give valid consent,

'it shall be lawful as being in the patient's best interests for the trust and/or the responsible medical practitioners having the responsibility at the time for the patient's treatment and care:

a to perform the said proposed gastrostomy;

b to withhold cardio-pulmonary resuscitation of the patient;

c to withhold the administration of antibiotics in the event of the patient developing a potentially life-threatening infection which would otherwise call for the administration of antibiotics but only if, immediately prior to the withholding of the same,

1 the trust is so advised both by the general medical practitioner and by the consultant psychiatrist having the responsibility at the time for the patient's treatment and care; and

2 one or other or both of the parents first give their consent thereto;

d generally to furnish such treatment and nursing care as may from time to time be appropriate to ensure that the patient suffers the least distress and retains the greatest dignity.'

Conclusion

The essential reason for euthanasia has always been that the victim's life is considered not worth living, whether by the doctor or nurse engaged in the acts or omissions causing the patient's death (whether or not the patient also regards their life as worthless) or by the relatives.

The Hippocratic tradition of avoidance of harm to the patient remains the principal ethical yardstick by which doctors should act (e.g in respect of CPR or DNR orders). The exception is that, with a court order, tube-feeding may lawfully be withdrawn from patients in PVS or near-PVS on the basis that it is not in their best interests to be so sustained. However, this exception granted by the law has not been without profound ethical problems. The withdrawal of hydration and nutrition from the non-dying patient is done in the knowledge that it will bring about the patient's death. As we have seen, it also requires tube-feeding to be regarded as treatment, rather than care, for a PVS patient when, in fact, it does not have a therapeutic effect but simply serves to keep the patient alive.

Keypoints

- Doctors are under an ethical duty not to kill their patients by act or omission.
- It is proper to withdraw futile treatments even if an earlier death is foreseen.
- Competent patients have a right to refuse treatment, but no right to commit suicide or to be assisted in suicide.
- Doctors should not intentionally assist suicidal refusals of treatment.
- Tube-feeding may lawfully be withdrawn from PVS patients, but only with a court order.

Chapter 13

Clinical research

Learning objectives

Core knowledge
- The nature and organization of clinical trials
- The ethical principles involved in human experimentation

Clinical Applications
- How to apply for ethical approval for a clinical trial
- Use of human organs and tissue

Background principles and case law
- Nuremberg War Crimes Trial ('The Doctors' Trial').
- Boundary between research and clinical practice
- Declaration of Helsinki

Introduction

Research is occasionally undertaken by medical students, but is usually first performed by a Specialist or Research Registrar when doing research towards a MD or Ph.D. Research is now less often seen as a requirement for career progression to Consultant, though it remains a requirement for academic medicine.

Students should understand the ethical principles involved in human experimentation and the conduct and organization of clinical trials. However, a detailed knowledge of how to submit a research ethics application is useful for anyone engaged in clinical research and sometimes for audit projects. The history of the development of research ethics following the Nuremberg War trials and the Declaration of Helsinki is of interest by way of background.

Nuremberg War Crimes Trial ('The Doctors' Trial')

The most famous medical trial in history was at Nuremberg after the Second World War, when 23 doctors were indicted by the International War Crimes Tribunal. Sixteen were found guilty. Seven were sentenced to death and were executed on 2 June 1948. A chilling account of the abuses of medicine and psychiatry under the Nazi regime can be read in Michael Burleigh's book *Death and Deliverance*.

The book gives a detailed description of the programme of euthanasia and forced sterilization, but also includes references to the stomach-churning 'medical' and 'scientific' experiments. Many of the perpetrators of these crimes escaped detection and punishment. There was even a 'defence' that such inhumane treatment of patients was not unique to doctors under the Nazi regimen (Table 13.1).

Following the Nuremberg Doctors' Trial, the War Crimes Tribunal laid down 10 standards to which physicians must conform when carrying out experiments on human subjects in the Nuremberg Code (Table 13.2). This formed the basis of the Declaration of Helsinki.

Table 13.1 Nuremberg Doctors' Trial. Were the Nazi atrocities unique?

> On 20 August 1945 Gerhard Rose, head of the department of tropical medicine at the Koch Institute, stood on trial at Nuremberg for 'murders, tortures, and other atrocities committed in the name of medical science'. At one point in the trial, Dr Rose and his defence counsel argued that the United States was guilty of similar medical practices, citing Dr Richard Strong, who had performed a series of studies in 1906 with 'cholera virus upon inmates of the Bilibid Prison in Manila'. Professor Strong later became Professor of Tropical Medicine at Harvard University. Another defendant at Nuremberg, Dr George Weltz, cited the case of another American doctor, Dr Joseph Goldberger, who induced pellagra in inmates of Rankin Farm Prison.
>
> Whilst these examples paled in comparison to the experiments perpetrated under the Nazis, American research relied heavily on prisoners during the Second World War. Examples include injections of blood from cattle as a source of plasma, atropine studies and experiments with sleeping sickness, sandfly fever, and dengue. One of the most widely publicized experiments during the War involved over 400 prisoners in malaria studies in Statesville Penitentiary in Illinois.

Table 13.2 Nuremberg Code 1947

> - The voluntary consent of the human subject is absolutely essential.
> - The experiment should be such as to yield fruitful results for the good of society that cannot be obtained by other means.
> - The anticipated results should justify the performance of the experiment.
> - The experiment should be conducted so as to avoid all unnecessary physical and mental suffering and injury.
> - No experiment should be performed when there is reason to believe that death or disabling injury may occur (except, perhaps, in those experiments where the experimenting physicians also serve as subjects).
> - The degree of risk should never exceed that determined by the humanitarian importance of the problem to be solved.
> - There should be adequate facilities to protect the subject against even remote possibilities of injury, disability or death.
> - The experiment should only be conducted by scientifically qualified persons, exercising the highest degree of skill and care throughout the experiment.
> - The subject should be at liberty to withdraw from the experiment.
> - The scientist in charge must be prepared to terminate the experiment if he has cause to believe that continuation is likely to cause injury to or death of the experimental subject.

Boundary between research and clinical practice

Research is essential for medicine to progress and develop. However the boundary between what is practice and what is research may, at times, be blurred. Generally 'practice' is taken to be anything done with the intention of producing a benefit to an individual patient within an everyday clinical setting. 'Research' usually means work done to test a hypothesis or to obtain or develop generalizable knowledge that may then be expressed as theories or principles. Clearly, there is considerable overlap between the two.

Not all practice is evidence-based, and much of what doctors do can be described as experimental in the sense of being new, untried or simply different. For example, drugs may be used by physicians to meet the needs of particular patients on a 'named patient basis' without being part of a for-mal research protocol. Indeed, research protocols may emerge because of chance findings in the response of patients to a particular drug or from general clinical experience. Without such serendipity many research opportunities would have been lost. For example, the immunosuppressive cyclosporin, which is routinely used after renal transplantation, may have a role in the management of fulminant ulcerative colitis in some patients. While clinical trials of cyclosporin in colitis have been conducted, one might ask whether the use of cyclosporin by a particular gastroenterologist in a particular patient who would otherwise be subject to a colectomy is research or clinical practice.

There are a number of problems and dangers that are intrinsic to medical research on human subjects:

- The outcome of the research is unknown—otherwise, the research would not be undertaken.
- Those participating are being 'used' as experimental subjects for the benefits of others, notwithstanding any benefits that directly or indirectly may accrue to themselves.
- Some experimental subjects are incapable of giving consent, e.g. children and the mentally incapacitated.
- There is risk of abuse, and exploitation of research subjects is not unknown.

An introduction to clinical trials

Clinical trials are at the heart of 'evidence-based medicine', and can be divided into:

- **Phase I studies**, which examine the safety and side-effects of new treatment either in patients or in healthy volunteers.
- **Phase II studies**, which aim to determine how effective the treatment is in patients with a particular condition.
- **Phase III studies**, which compare the treatment with the best currently available treatment, or with placebo where there is no effective therapy.

Care must be taken when trials are placebo-controlled and there is a 'no treatment' control group. These can usually only be justified if there is no currently effective therapy available, or if the condition is minor and the patients receiving placebo will not be subject to any appreciable risk of harm (Table 13.3).

Ethical issues in research using human subjects

The ethical principles underlying clinical research and based largely on the Nuremberg Code were updated by the World Health Organization in the 2000 version of the Declaration of Helsinki. A summary of the fundamental ethical principles is given in Table 13.4.

There are a number of ethical considerations when human subjects participate in clinical research. The main priority is the safety of the participant, which requires a careful analysis of the risks and benefits of the research. This is particu-

Table 13.3 Use of placebo-controlled trials

The benefits, risks, burdens and effectiveness of a new method should be tested against those of the best current prophylactic, diagnostic, and therapeutic methods. This does not exclude the use of placebo, or no treatment, in studies where no proven prophylactic, diagnostic or therapeutic method exists.

However, a placebo-controlled trial may be ethically acceptable, even if proven therapy is available, under the following circumstances:
- Where for compelling and scientifically sound methodological reasons its use is necessary to determine the efficacy or safety of a prophylactic, diagnostic or therapeutic method; or
- Where a prophylactic, diagnostic or therapeutic method is being investigated for a minor condition and the patients who receive placebo will not be subject to any additional risk of serious or irreversible harm.

Declaration of Helsinki 2002, amendment to paragraph 29.

larly important when the subjects are healthy volunteers or where the research is non-therapeutic. The safety of the individual is less of an issue in observational compared to interventional studies. The investigator must consider how adverse events will be handled and compensation will be provided.

The investigator must obtain informed consent and ensure privacy and confidentiality of information from unauthorized access. Subjects may wish to know the results of the research and any personal information that may be of importance to them that may have been discovered during the course of the trial.

In designing and executing the trial the investigator must be in a state of 'equipoise', that is, a state of genuine uncertainty as to the outcome. A true 'null hypothesis' should be tested, namely that there is no known difference between the proposed treatment and the currently best available treatment or no treatment, where conventional therapy is ineffective.

All research must be founded on the three principles of respect for persons, beneficence and justice.

Table 13.4 Ethical principles in human research

- **Respect for persons**
  'It is the duty of the physician in medical research to protect the life, health, privacy, and dignity of the human subject.'
- **Requirement for informed consent to research**
  'Subjects must be volunteers and informed participants in the research project.'
- **Beneficence**
  'In medical research on human subjects, considerations related to the well-being of the human subject should take precedence over the interests of science and society.'
- **Justice**
  — **research should be directed primarily towards meeting the needs of patients rather than commercial interests**
  'The researcher should also submit to the [ethics] committee, for review, information regarding funding, sponsors, institutional affiliations, other potential conflicts of interest and incentives for subjects.'
  — **those who take part in research should also be potential beneficiaries of the research**
  'At the conclusion of the study, every patient entered into the study should be assured of access to the best proven prophylactic, diagnostic and therapeutic methods identified by the study.'
  — **research should not be conducted on subject groups unlikely ever to benefit from the results**
  'Medical research is only justified if there is a reasonable likelihood that the population in which the research is carried out stand to benefit from the results of the research.'

Respect for persons

According to the Declaration of Helsinki:

'Medical research is subject to ethical standards that promote respect for all human beings and protect their health and rights.'

'It is the duty of the physician in medical research to protect the life, health, privacy, and dignity of the human subject.'

Respect for persons requires recognition of personal autonomy, integrity, privacy and confidentiality. Care must be taken to protect those who are open to coercion and undue influence. This applies particularly to the vulnerable, prisoners, those in institutional care and anyone in a dependent relationship to the investigator.

Requirement for informed consent to research

Fully informed consent is an ethical requirement for therapeutic research, since the subjects are agreeing to interventions that are not required for routine medical care. The 'therapeutic privilege' does not apply. The subjects must be fully informed about the trial, with such information including the nature and purpose of the research, the procedures involved, particularly if they involve risk (including risks from ionizing radiation), and the possible benefits to the individual and to society. The subjects must be given time to ensure that they understand the study, and must have time to ask questions. They must also understand that in the case of therapeutic research they can withdraw and that this would not prejudice their routine medical care. In the case of non-intervention studies in patients and volunteer studies, there is also a need for full disclosure of the nature and purpose of the research. By giving consent to the research the subject does not waive any legal rights or release the investigator from liability for negligence.

All consent to research must be voluntary, free from any coercion or undue influence. According to the Declaration of Helsinki:

'When obtaining informed consent for the research project the physician should be particularly cautious if the subject is in a dependent relationship with the physician or may consent under duress. In that case the informed consent should be obtained by a well-informed physician who is not engaged in the investigation and who is completely independent of this relationship.'

Declaration of Helsinki 2002

Beneficence

'It is the duty of the physician to promote and safeguard the health of the people. The physician's knowledge and conscience are dedicated to the fulfilment of this duty.'

'Consideration of the well-being of the subject must take precedence over the interests of science and society.'

Declaration of Helsinki 2002

Beneficence requires that benefits should be maximized and harm minimized. All research must weight the potential benefits to the participants against risks. The study should be stopped if the risks are found to outweigh the benefits or where there is no conclusive proof of positive and beneficial results. This may result in an early termination of the trial.

Justice

Medicine has enormous potential not only to benefit humanity but also for crimes against humanity, particularly, though not exclusively, in the course of human experimentation. The Nuremberg Code had a profound effect on human experimentation. Nevertheless, the 'Doctors' Trial' emphasized how the medical profession should exercise its healing functions for those vulnerable people who seek care and treatment. Many fundamental issues of justice were raised at Nuremberg that remain relevant today, including the relationship between the physician and the State in the face of institutional brutality and discrimination.

Considerations of justice apply to the selection of research topics as well as subjects for research. It is important not to discriminate against particular classes of individuals, e.g. those from particular racial or ethnic groups, or the disabled. Certain illnesses attract more academic attention and funding than others. Compare, for example, research into dementia versus cardiac research, or cancer research in developed countries against infectious diseases in developing countries. Research should not unduly involve groups who are unlikely to benefit from the subsequent developments in medical practice.

Research Ethics committees

European Union Clinical Trials directive

In May 2001 the European Union Clinical Trials Directive was issued (Directive 2001/20/EC) and implemented in UK domestic law in May 2004.

The Directive covers all interventional studies that have been registered with the Department of Health, whether sponsored by the Research Councils, charitable organizations, industry, professional bodies, NHS Trusts, health authorities, government departments or universities. No distinction is made between commercial and non-commercial trials. The Directive also covers healthy volunteer studies. The Directive provides for the protection of human subjects, including minors and incapacitated adults.

The Directive will:

• establish ethics committees on a legal basis;
• lay down standards for the investigation of the manufacture, import and labelling of medicinal products;
• provide for quality assurance and safety monitoring of clinical trials;
• require that investigators have a clinical trial authorization (CTA).

The EU Directive will have a significant impact on the conduct of clinical trials, including a financial impact.

Working arrangements and governance of NHS Research Ethics Committees

All research on human subjects must be assessed and agreed with a research ethics committee (REC). This is both an ethical requirement under the Declaration of Helsinki and a legal requirement, particularly in the light of the vigorous standards set by the European Directive 2001. All RECs are independent bodies and are not accountable to NHS trusts.

Research Ethics Committees are divided into Local (LREC) and Multi-centre (MREC) Research Ethics Committees (LRECs and MRECs). LRECs are appointed by the Health Authority. MRECs are appointed by the Department of Health, and cover five or more 'sites', defined as the geographical areas of the respective Health Authorities. Normally decisions are required from MRECs concerning the overall ethical acceptability of the trial before the issue is devolved to the LRECs, which will then decide 'locality' issues.

Once approval is gained from the MREC, the 'locality issues' decided by the LREC are restricted to:
• the suitability of the local researcher, e.g. qualifications and experience;
• the appropriateness of the local research environment and facilities, e.g. disruption of services and issues of workload;
• specific issues relating to the local community, e.g. the need to provide information, e.g. in languages other than English.

The Department of Health has also set up additional ethics committees for specialist areas, including the Gene Therapy Advisory Committee (GTAC), the United Kingdom Xenotransplantation Regulatory Authority (UKXIRA) and the Human Fertilization and Embryology Authority (HFEA).

The Central Office for Research Ethics Committees (COREC) works on behalf of the Department of Health to co-ordinate, review and develop the work of RECs, and sets out general principles and operating standards.

Remit of an NHS REC

Authorization from an NHS REC is required for any research involving:
• patients and users of the NHS or persons identified as potential participants because of their status as relatives or carers of NHS patients;
• access to data, organs or tissues of past and present NHS patients;
• foetal material and IVF using NHS patients;
• the recently dead in NHS premises;
• use of NHS premises or facilities; or
• NHS staff.

MRECs cover multi-centre research at five or more sites, defined as the geographical area of a single Health Authority.

Membership requirements

The Health Authority is responsible for appointing LREC members and the Department of Health for members of MRECs. Appointments should be according to Nolan principles, and are usually for 5 years, but not for more than two consecutive 5-year terms. COREC recommends that membership of a REC should be recognized in job plans. Appointed members should be prepared to publish their full name, profession, affiliations and interests. A condition of appointment is to participate in training and continued education. Members are bound by confidentiality. Legal liability for actions taken by members of RECs is taken by the appointing authority except for bad faith, wilful default or gross negligence, which are not covered.

RECs should normally have a maximum of 18 members, with a mixture of expert and lay members, so that the scientific, clinical, methodological and wider ethical and welfare implications of the research can be fully assessed.

Expert members should be chosen to have a range of expertise in:
• clinical and non-clinical research methodology;
• statistics relevant to research;
• clinical practice in both a hospital and a community setting; and
• pharmacy.

At least one-third of the committee membership should be 'lay' members, who should be independent of the NHS and whose primary personal or professional interests should not be in research. Lay members may include non-medical clinic staff who have not practised for at least 5 years.

Specialist referees as non-voting members of the committee may occasionally be required to review particular projects.

A quorum will normally consist of seven members, including the Chair/Vice Chair, an expert and a lay member, and at least one member who is independent of the institution.

Working procedures of RECs

REC working practices must now be compatible with European and UK law and conform to ethical standards set by professional bodies such as the Medical Research Council.

Research Ethics Councils should:
- make decisions at scheduled meetings at which a quorum is present;
- meet regularly—usually every month;
- retain records for at least 3 years after completion of the research;
- provide timely advice, usually within 60 days of the first application. However, where substantial amendments are required a further application may be required within the standard 60-day timeframe;
- require progress and final reports from the researcher;
- issue an annual report to the appointing Authority. The responsibilities of the researcher to the REC are to:
- provide full information regarding the trial;
- notify any changes of protocol to the REC;
- provide interim progress reports, e.g. annually and in a final report;
- report any major adverse events or unusual or unexpected side-effects that might affect the safety of trial participants;
- Early termination of the trial should also be notified to the REC, with reasons.

The process of ethical review by Research Ethics committees

A number of elements need to be considered by a REC before giving ethical approval, as is shown in Table 13.5.

The process of ethical review by REC

The primary role of the REC is to determine whether the research proposal meets acceptable ethical standards, particularly in relation to:
- patient safety
- informed consent
- quality of the study and chances of producing useful results
- suitability and feasibility of the protocol
- any relevant laws and regulations, e.g. EU Directives.

Table 13.5 Factors to be considered in a research application

- Has a systematic review of the literature been undertaken?
- What is the problem to be addressed?
- What is the hypothesis to be tested? What are the primary and secondary outcome measures?
- Will the results genuinely contribute to new knowledge of the subject or advances in diagnosis or treatment?
- How will the results of the trial be used?
- What are the safety issues for participants?
- What type of study is involved, e.g. interventional, or observational, and what is the study design, e.g. is it a double-blind placebo trial?
- What is the expected duration of the trial and what are the inclusion and exclusion criteria?
- How will patients be recruited, e.g. by use of patient databases or public advertisements? What is the expected recruitment rate?
- Is it of sufficient statistical power to give meaningful results, and has statistical advice been sought during the design of the trial?
- Will there be any factors that might put at risk the completion of the study, e.g. patient numbers, costs, equipment? Was there a pilot study to assess feasibility?
- What are the specific interventions—e.g. radiological investigations, drug treatment or other diagnostic or therapeutic procedures—and what are the risks?
- Will women of reproductive age be included in the study, and, if so, how will they be protected?
- What are the proposed benefits of the study?
- Will the participants be informed of the results?
- Is the opportunity to use/not use any beneficial treatment made clear to the patients, e.g. by continuation of a drug on a 'named patient' basis?
- What are the arrangements to protect patient confidentiality?
- What are the arrangements for data storage? (Normally research data should be made available for reference or verification purposes for at least 10 years after the study, or longer if required by a research body.)
- How will patients be allocated to treatment groups? What are the randomization procedures?
- Are the patient information leaflets sufficiently clear? Is there any possibility of undue influence or conflict of interest in the recruitment of patients?
- Are there suitable arrangements to contact the investigators in the event of adverse events, or if it is

Table 13.5 *Continued*

necessary, to break randomization codes or discontinue treatment?
● Will the patient's GP be informed of the study?
● Are there likely to be any particular problems with compliance?
● Are there suitable arrangements for no-fault compensation? How are the investigators indemnified?

Table 13.6 Embryo research permitted by law

Research is permitted on embryos under HFEA Act 1990 to advance knowledge or pursue developments in the following areas:
● fertility treatment
● congenital disease
● miscarriages
● contraception
● pre-implantation genetic diagnosis.
In January 2001 the Government added the following indications:
● embryonic development
● serious disease
● treatments for serious disease.

The REC is primarily concerned with the protection of human subjects involved in clinical research. Unscientific studies of poor quality that are unlikely to produce meaningful or useful results are therefore unethical. Studies that are not feasible, with poor chances of reaching completion though lack of resources or poor recruitment of patients are also unethical. Human research ought to be of publishable quality.

Human cloning for research purposes ('research cloning')

'Therapeutic cloning' is the term to describe what is, in effect, cloning for the purposes of research. The term 'research cloning' is less ambiguous than 'therapeutic cloning'. At the time of writing, cloned human embryos have not been put to direct therapeutic use. However, embryonic nerve cells have been used to treat patients with Parkinson's disease. The HFEA Act 1990 specifically prohibits keeping or using an embryo after the appearance of the primitive streak or after 14 days, whichever is the earlier. The placement of a human embryo in a non-human animal and altering the genetic structure of any cell whilst it forms a part of an embryo are both prohibited by law.

Embryo research is permitted by law under the HFEA Act 1990 (and the 2001 Regulations) for the reasons shown in Table 13.6.

The use of human organs and tissue: an interim report (DOH April 2003)

Present law on the removal, retention and use of human tissues and organs contains many uncer-

tainties, particularly after the Alder Hey scandal (Table 13.7).

The Department of Health issued interim guidelines on the use of human organs and tissues in April 2003.

Human tissues and organs may be used for:
● post mortem examination to establish the cause of death
● training, education and research
● public health surveillance
● organ transplantation
● transplantation of tissues or cells, e.g. marrow transplants
● blood transfusions
● use of foetal tissue in research and for other purposes, e.g. the development of vaccines
● tissue engineering, e.g. to produce substitute skin, bone or cartilage.

Recommendations on the removal of tissues and organs from living patients

The human body and its parts should be treated with respect, and before removal of tissues or organs patients:
● should be provided with appropriate information about the reasons for the removal and the use to which the material will be put;
● should have the opportunity to ask questions and give valid consent;
● must consent voluntarily without any undue pressure.

Table 13.7 The Alder Hey Inquiry

The inquiry was established in December 1999 following evidence to the Bristol Inquiry that a large number of hearts from deceased children were retained in NHS hospitals.

In addition to hearts other organs were also retained at the Alder Hey Hospital without consent.

Professor Van Velzen, the Chair of Foetal and Infant Pathology, was accused of unethically and illegally taking organs from children at post mortem. Most of the organs taken were not used for medical research. Complaints were made by parents that their children had not been buried intact. Some parents faced up to four funerals as parts were returned to them. Professor Van Veltzen was later suspended by the GMC. As a result of the Inquiry the Rt Hon. Alan Milburn MP, the Secretary of State, said in Parliament:

'The NHS can no longer assume that the benefits of science, medicine or research are somehow self-evident regardless of the wishes of patients or their families. The relationship between patients and the service today has to be based on informed consent. That will require changes in practice and changes in policy. It will require changes in medical education. As I have made clear today it will also require changes to the law.'

In February 2003 some 1,154 complainants received £5 million in an out-of-court settlement for the Alder Hey scandal.

On 3 December 2003 the Government introduced the Human Tissue Bill, which would criminalize the removal of body parts without consent, with a maximum penalty of a prison sentence of 12 months. It also proposes to set up the Human Tissue Authority, with a remit to grant licences for anatomical examinations of bodies, post mortems and the storage and use of body parts.

Material taken at post mortem

A coroner's post mortem does not require consent. However, consent should be sought for the retention of tissues or organs after the Coroner no longer has any use for them (unless retention is required by the Police and Criminal Evidence Act 1984). Where there is a hospital post mortem and the deceased has not expressed any wishes with re-gard to the retention of tissues or organs, consent should be sought from the person closest to the deceased. According to the Department of Health, this is the only way that the requirements of the Human Tissue Act 1961 can be met.

Research using tissue or organs

Tissue or organs should be used in research only if the benefits outweigh any potential harm to the donor of the tissue and the research is approved by a properly constituted ethics committee. Samples of tissues or organs obtained for research should be regarded as donations, and the use of such material should not, as such, lead to overall financial gain. However, it would be legitimate to levy certain administrative or handling charges. Furthermore, it would also be legitimate for those who develop new products from the use of such material to 'seek a financial return for their skills and labour'. Research participants should know, if they wish, individual research results that may affect their interests.

It may sometimes be difficult to know in the case of stored material whether consent to the use of tissue and organs for research has been properly obtained. Where appropriate, consent ought to be obtained from the person concerned, or, where he cannot be traced, or has died, from a person close to him or her. It cannot be assumed that stored material has simply been 'abandoned'. However, obtaining consent may involve undue distress, and the Retained Organs Commission has suggested that families who have no prior knowledge of organ retention should not be contacted about the post mortem use of material for research. The use of unidentified material is not necessarily unethical. Nevertheless, it is important to distinguish between material obtained surgically and at post mortem.

On the basis largely of MRC recommendations the Department of Health suggests that the following stipulations should govern the use of unidentified surgical specimens:
• That the project is approved by a research ethics committee.
• That there is no potential harm to donors.

• That preference should be given to the use of tissue for which valid consent has been obtained over that where the circumstances of the consent are inadequately documented.

• That the material has not been obtained in an unethical manner, and there are no cultural objections to its use.

Other uses of human tissues or organs

Tissues or organs may also be used in a number of other contexts, including:

• in-service training
• quality assurance and audit
• formal education
• public health surveillance
• laboratory tests.

Tissues and organs may be used for postgraduate and undergraduate teaching, courses and in-service training. It is recommended that there should be arrangements for informing patients that material may be used for these purposes. If a patient opts out this should be respected. Consent for the use of material is not necessary where in-service training is part of normal clinical practice. Patients have a right not to allow samples to be used in surveys or to be used in the assessment or improvement of laboratory tests.

Part 5

Maintaining Standards and Professional Regulation

Maintaining standards and professional regulation

Learning objectives

Core knowledge
- Existing legislation regarding professional regulation
- Organizational changes within the NHS to improve healthcare delivery
- The role of the GMC
- Duties of a doctor as defined by the GMC

Practical applications
- Continuing professional development
- Clinical governance

Background principles
- Educational or punitive models of accountability

Introduction

Medical mishaps and serious adverse events are a fact of medical practice. It is no longer true to say that junior doctors will not be called upon at Coroner's inquests or face civil claims in negligence (Table 14.1). The naming and shaming of doctors in the press is no longer reserved for Consultants. It is important to have some understanding of how complaints procedures are handled by the NHS and a background understanding of risk-management strategies.

The cumulative cost of adverse events to the NHS and the economy is massive (Table 14.2).

However, disciplinary proceedings are often time-consuming, protracted and stressful for doctors, and have led to depression and even suicide.

A basic understanding of the way that the medical profession is regulated is important for all doctors, who are now required to be regularly revalidated in order to maintain their registration to practice. The pre-registration year enables the newly qualified doctor to develop the professional skills required of a registered medical practitioner under supervision. The acquisition of such professional skills is still based upon an apprenticeship model.

The important message from this Chapter is that professional regulation is here to stay. There are a number of recent organizational changes in place both within the NHS and GMC to make it a practical reality.

A profession is a group of individuals who share particular knowledge and skills and are bound by a common code of conduct. The medical profession is regulated both by the General Medical Council and by a number of disciplinary processes and NHS complaints procedures. We begin by considering the various mechanisms for regulation of doctors and other healthcare professionals within the NHS before considering the role of the General Medical Council. GMC procedures will be dealt with in detail in Chapter 17.

Table 14.1 Gross failure by a SHO to recognize post-operative haemorrhage

A 42-year-old woman died as a result of a post-operative haemorrhage after a hysterectomy under an epidural anaesthetic. The SHO had thought that hypotension was due to the epidural rather than to a haemorrhage, and had not summoned help until it was too late.

A Consultant Gynaecologist commented that: 'This was clearly a preventable death. All the signs were there that it was a haemorrhage that was causing hypotension, and a senior consultant or anaesthetist would have immediately recognized them.'

The Coroner recorded a verdict of 'death by misadventure, to which neglect contributed' and criticized the hospital's 'gross failure to provide basic medical care'.

It can no longer be assumed that junior doctors will not be held to account for clinical errors. The fact that the SHO had only worked in the Department for 10 days was not an extenuating circumstance.

Reported in *The Times*, 4 February 2004

Table 14.2 Epidemiology and cost of adverse medical events

Every year:
- adverse events occur in around 10% of admissions—or in excess of 850,000 per year
- cost the health service an estimated £2 billion in additional hospital stays
- 400 people die or are seriously injured in adverse events involving medical devices
- nearly 10,000 people are reported to have experienced serious adverse reactions to drugs
- around 1,150 people who have been in recent contact with mental health services commit suicide
- hospital-acquired infections—around 15% of which may be avoidable—are estimated to cost the NHS nearly £1 billion
- the NHS pays out around £400 million in settlement of clinical negligence claims.

An Organization with a Memory: Report of an Expert Group on Learning From Adverse Events in the NHS. Chaired by the Chief Medical Officer. DoH (2000).

A new and often unfamiliar vocabulary has sprung up in relation to many of the subjects discussed in this chapter. For definitions and explanations of terms please see the Glossary at the end of Chapter 15. Appendix 5 lists some of the relevant Acts that form the legislative framework of the NHS.

The Bristol Inquiry

The Bristol Inquiry was set up by the Health Secretary Mr Frank Dobson to investigate children's heart surgery at the Bristol Royal Infirmary from 1984 to 1995 after an unacceptably high mortality was uncovered. As a result of the 'Bristol scandal' Mr Wisheart and Dr Roylance were struck off the medical register and Dr Dhasmana was censured by the GMC. The Inquiry was empowered to investigate the adequacy of services, including any professional, managerial and organizational failures and the measures taken to deal with concerns raised about paediatric cardiac surgery.

Some key recommendations of the Inquiry are outlined in Table 14.3.

Models of accountability: educational or punitive?

Two models for professional accountability have been proposed—the educational and the punitive.

The educational model regards mistakes as learning opportunities, and assumes that if there is a spirit of openness ('no blame culture') people will be willing to admit their failings and learn from their mistakes. The punitive model aims to punish those who make mistakes as a means of compensation for the victims, as a form of retribution and as a means of deterrence to prevent mistakes from arising in the future.

While few would disagree with the educational model, there must also be a punitive element for reckless behaviour and incompetence. However, the punitive model may tempt people to conceal their mistakes. Both systems require reporting of critical incidents to employers who also have

Table 14.3 Some key recommendations of the Bristol Inquiry

- A culture within the NHS which promotes greater openness, accountability, flexibility and multidisciplinary teamwork
- Greater emphasis on patient safety and the quality of care.
- Incentives for critical incident-reporting, such as providing immunity for those reporting adverse events.
- Abolition of the current clinical negligence system as part of the 'culture of blame', and consideration of no-blame compensation.
- Respect and honesty towards patients. Greater patient involvement in treatment decisions and a duty of candour when things go wrong.
- A well-led health service with improved management at all levels.
- Competent healthcare professionals with up-to-date knowledge and skills.
- Care of an appropriate standard, informed by current knowledge and best practice.
- Guaranteed generic standards for healthcare institutions through regular external inspection and validation.
- Public involvement through empowerment in the planning, organization and delivery of healthcare.

Table 14.4 Possible developments in professional regulation

- Place greater emphasis on education and training.
- Achieve an accurate delineation of punishable issues.
- Doctors might be encouraged to report mistakes if granted a degree of immunity (Bristol).
- Create no-fault compensation schemes.
- Create a 'blame-free' and 'patient safety' culture through risk management.
- Separate organizations with an educational role from those with a disciplinary/punishment function.
- Ensure that education and training should not be too time-consuming, and that the benefits are apparent.

disciplinary powers. At present the confidentiality arrangements and guidance as to the immunities (if any) granted to those reporting mistakes are still being worked out. It is hoped that appraisal may have a role in identifying those whose performance is poor.

Appraisal is now a contractual requirement, and will form the basis of revalidation by the GMC. New educational initiatives are in place in the form of continuous professional development (CPD), which is an extension of continuous medical education (CME). Nevertheless, there has been an expansion of punitive measures against doctors, and a new body, the Council For Regulation of Health Care Professionals, has been set up with an overarching responsibility for all healthcare professionals and powers to challenge unduly lenient decisions of the GMC. Some possible approaches to the roles of education and punishment in professional regulation are suggested in Table 14.4.

NHS complaints procedures

In 1998/9 there were 86,000 written complaints against hospital and community health services in England, with 1,800 requests for independent review, 39,000 complaints against family health services and 1,430 requests for independent review. Hence, between 96% and 98% of complaints do not proceed beyond the initial stages.

All complaints procedures, whether against hospital doctors, GPs, or NHS organizations, have three stages in common:
- Local Review
- Independent Review
- Appeal to the Health Service Commissioner (popularly called the Ombudsman), who can investigate all aspects of the complaint, including the clinical aspects.

Organizational changes to improve healthcare delivery

The NHS Complaints procedures address complaints against individual doctors and nurses. In recent years there have been various Government initiatives, backed up by legislation, to examine and improve healthcare standards at an organizational level. At the heart of this approach lie clinical governance, annual appraisal and GMC revalidation.

Clinical governance

The Government's white paper *A First Class Service* defined clinical governance as:

'a framework through which NHS organizations are accountable for continuously improving the quality of their services and safeguarding high standards of care by creating an environment in which excellence in clinical care will flourish.'

Clinical Governance covers a range of strategies to monitor and improve standards, including:
- clinical risk management
- clinical audit
- continuing professional development (CPD)
- annual appraisal and regular review of job plans for consultants
- regular revalidation of doctors
- National Service Frameworks
- National Institute of Clinical Effectiveness (NICE) Guidelines
- inspections of NHS Trusts by the Commission for Health Care Audit and Inspection (CHAI).

The Chief Executive must identify a lead clinician, who is not necessarily a doctor, who will be responsible to the relevant NHS Board for clinical governance.

Table 14.5 Risk management standards set by the clinical negligence scheme for trusts

- Written strategy on clinical risk management
- Clinical reporting system
- Rapid follow-up of major incidents
- Agreed system for managing complaints
- Appropriate information for patients regarding treatment
- Adequate record-keeping and audit of medical records
- Systems for ensuring clinical competence and training of staff
- Clinical risk-management system in place
- Procedures for management of general clinical care
- System for management and communication in maternity care
- Public and patient protection in mental health services

Clinical risk management

The purpose of clinical risk management is to examine, monitor and advise on matters that may lead to harm to patients. NHS boards are required to have a written strategy for risk management, with clear lines of responsibility and accountability. The Clinical Negligence Scheme for Trusts introduced standards for NHS Trusts regarding risk management (Table 14.5).

Clinical audit

Clinical audit is a systematic critical analysis of the quality of health care. The aim of audit is to identify and implement opportunities for improvement against set standards based upon best available evidence of good clinical practice. The 'audit cycle' is completed by revisiting the subject and demonstrating improvements. Unlike other forms of audit, clinical audit does not have a financial focus. Participation in audit is a mandatory requirement for appraisal and revalidation for doctors.

National regulatory bodies

Department of Health: National Service Frameworks (NSF)

National Service Frameworks set national standards and outline strategies for service implementation within particular clinical areas. They also define performance milestones and time-scales. A rolling programme of NSFs was begun in 1998, and to date includes cancer, paediatric intensive care, mental health, coronary heart disease, diabetes, renal services and care of the elderly. Each National Service Framework is developed with external reference groups, bringing together professionals, service-users and carers, partner agencies and health-service managers. The overall process is managed by the Department of Health.

National Institute for Clinical Excellence (NICE)

The National Institute for Clinical Excellence was set up in April 1999 as a Special Health Authority under s.11 of the National Health Service Act 1977. NICE provides patients, healthcare professionals and the public with authoritative guidance on current best clinical practice. It provides advice on the clinical effectiveness and cost-effectiveness of new technology, drugs, devices, diagnostic techniques and therapeutic procedures, and issues guidelines on the clinical management of specific diseases.

In November 2002, 30 lay members were elected to a new Citizens Council to reflect public opinion in the guidance that NICE publishes about the clinical effectiveness and cost-effectiveness of treatments for the NHS.

Commission for Health Improvement (CHI)

CHI was established to improve the quality of care for patients in England and Wales. In Scotland the corresponding body is the Clinical Standards Board.

CHI has four statutory functions:
- To review clinical governance.
- To monitor and review the application of NSF and NICE guidelines.
- To investigate serious failures in the NHS.
- To lead, review and assist NHS healthcare improvements.

CHI works closely with the Department of Health, but is independent of it. There are plans to extend the remit of CHI to review all aspects of patient care and publish a range of information about the NHS, including performance ratings (league tables) and the outcomes of NSF studies. From November 2002, under the terms of the Freedom of Information Act 2000, CHI provides a comprehensive list of documents that are available to the public.

CHI focuses on systems and processes at an organizational level, and not on the performance of individuals.

The National Health Service Reform and Health Care Professions Act 2002 ('the 2002 Act') extends the role of CHI and enables it to discharge its responsibilities relating to the collection and analysis of data and performance assessment through the Office for Information in Health Care Performance. The 2002 Act also widens the powers of CHI to inspect service-providers and recommend to the Secretary of State that special remedial measures be taken when services are of an unacceptably poor standard.

Commission for Health Care Audit and Inspection (CHAI)

The remit of CHAI now encompasses:
- all the current and proposed work of CHI and the Mental Health Act Commission and
- the work of the Audit Commission in relation to value-for-money work in the NHS and
- independent healthcare work of the National Care Standards Commission.

National Patient Safety Agency (NPSA)

The NPSA is a Special Health Authority created in July 2001 to co-ordinate efforts around the country to report and learn from adverse events occurring in the NHS. It aims to promote an open and fair culture in hospitals and to encourage doctors to report incidents without fear of reprisal.

Patients' forums

The 2002 Act establishes Patient Forums, which may provide a lay input into the setting up and running of medical services and involvement in independent complaints advocacy, and can provide advice to patients and carers about local complaints procedures.

Commission for Patient and Public Involvement in Health (CPPIH)

The CPPIH was established as an independent corporate body under the 2002 Act to advise the Secretary of State on the involvement of patients and the public regarding matters concerning health service. The CPPIH may investigate and report on matters that may, for example, be brought to its attention by a Patients' Forum, CHAI, the NPSA or National Care Standards Commission. The CPPIH will promote public involvement in health care at a national level, while Patients' Forums will do so at a local level.

Focus on the performance of individuals

Continuing professional development (CPD)

'CPD is a process of lifelong systematic learning for all individuals and teams which enables them to meet the needs of patients and to deliver the health outcomes and healthcare priorities of the NHS or other employers and which enables professionals to expand and fulfil their potential.'

Academy of Medical Royal Colleges, 1998

CPD is now a requirement for doctors who have completed their higher specialist training or obtained a permanent position in hospital or general practice. It replaces continuing medical education (or CME). It is now recognized that CPD should cover a range of activities that extends beyond simply attending courses and conferences. These additional activities include obtaining further qualifications, learning new skills and gaining experience in areas related to clinical practice, such as management and medical law.

Annual appraisal

Annual appraisal is now a contractual requirement for consultants and GPs to assess their performance and career development. Appraisal for Consultants was launched in April 2001 and for GPs in April 2002. Periodic review has always been a requirement for trainees. Appraisal involves a constructive dialogue with a professional peer, e.g. a clinical or medical director. Appraisal will form part of revalidation and ongoing registration with the GMC, and assesses an individual's work using comparative performance data from local, regional and national sources. It provides an opportunity for the appraisees to identify their professional and service needs, resource issues, development opportunities and service requirements. It can also be used to review participation in wider NHS activities such as research, teaching, college work and involvement with national bodies such as the GMC.

Revalidation

Revalidation will mean that a doctor's licence to practice will need to be renewed every five years. Ongoing registration will indicate that the doctor is recognized by the GMC as fit to practise medicine by complying with defined professional standards, keeping up to date and maintaining clinical competence. For most doctors annual appraisal will provide suitable evidence for revalidation. Doctors who choose not to participate in revalidation will lose the right to exercise the privileges of registration.

Doctors will be asked for evidence under the seven headings set out in the GMC guidance *Good Medical Practice*:

- Good clinical care
- Maintaining good medical practice
- Teaching and training
- Relationships with patients
- Working with colleagues
- Probity
- Health.

Instructions for revalidation were issued by the GMC in 2003.

Disciplinary procedures for general practitioners

The Health and Social Care Act 2001 abolished the NHS Tribunal, which had powers to suspend or disqualify general practitioners. New powers of disciplinary action were devolved to Health Authorities as a transitional arrangement before Primary Care Trusts (in England) took on these roles between April 2002 and 2003. The position in Wales is under review, as Welsh Health Authorities will be abolished in March 2003.

• **Family Health Services Appeal Authority (FHSAA)**

The FHSAA was set up by The Family Health Services Appeal Authority (Primary Care Act) Regulations 2001. The FHSAA inherit the role of the NHS Tribunal to decide on the right of return of a doctor to the General Medical Services (GMS) list and hence GMS practice.

• **Local Medical Committee (LMC)**

A statutory representative body elected by GPs in a defined geographical area. LMCs pre-date the NHS and have existed in much the same form since 1911. Statutory health organizations are required by NHS Regulations to consult the LMC on a variety of general medical service issues. The medical secretary or chair of an LMC can be a key contact when dealing with doctors who are causing concern. LMCs are represented nationally by the General Practitioners Committee (GPC) of the British Medical Association (BMA). The LMC can give advice to practitioners over a wide range of issues including disputes between partners, contractual matters and the handling of complaints. Where necessary, the LMC may represent practitioners who are the subject of Independent Reviews or disciplinary procedures.

• **National Clinical Assessment Authority (NCAA)**

This is a Special Health Authority established as one of the central elements of the NHS programme on quality. It started work in April 2001 and provides support to Health Authorities and Primary Care, Hospital and Community Trusts when they are faced with concerns over the performance of individual doctors. The NCAA will not take over the role of employer nor act as a regulator. However, it will help the employer or Health Authority to carry out an objective assessment, after which it will advise on the appropriate course of action. The involvement of lay people is an important aspect of the service.

Statutory regulation of professional standards: the role of the GMC

The General Medical Council (GMC) is a statutory body that was first set up under the Medical Act of 1858. It continues to regulate the medical profession under the Medical Act 1983, as amended. The main role of the GMC is to protect patients from bad medical practice, and its motto is 'protecting patients, guiding doctors'. While the GMC cannot decide cases or issue advice that is contrary to the civil or criminal law, its views and guidelines will be influential in determining what constitutes ethical conduct. Moreover, it may declare a practice unethical that is not technically illegal, e.g. the advertising of medical services (although this has been somewhat relaxed in recent years). It also has statutory powers to censure or erase doctors from the medical register for professional misconduct.

Major reforms of the GMC took place in 2002/3 to take account of revalidation and to modify its procedures. The regulatory procedures of the GMC are dealt with in Chapter 17.

The National Health Service Reform and Health Care Professions Act 2002 set up an overarching council for all healthcare professionals known as the Council for the Regulation of Health Care Professionals, which can investigate the performance of any of the regulatory bodies such as the GMC. The number of complaints against doctors made to the GMC has shown a steady rise in recent years (Table 14.6).

Responsibilities of the GMC

The GMC has four main statutory responsibilities:
• Maintaining standards of medical education
• Keeping a register of doctors deemed fit to practise (the Medical Register)

Table 14.6 Complaints made to the GMC

YEAR	Total number of complaints
1995	1503
1997	2687
2000	4470
2001	4504

Handling the 4,500 complaints made against doctors in 2001 cost £18.8m, or £4,000 per complaint.

- Taking disciplinary action against doctors, including erasure from the Register
- Providing advice on professional standards and medical ethics.

Duties of a doctor registered with the general medical council

The professional duties of doctors were outlined by the GMC in 1998:

'Patients must be able to trust doctors with their lives and well-being. To justify that trust, we as a profession have a duty to maintain a good standard of practice and care to show respect for human life. In particular as a doctor you must:
- Make the care of your patient your first concern.
- Treat every patient politely and considerately.
- Respect patients' dignity and privacy.
- Listen to patients and respect their views.
- Give patients information in a way they can understand.
- Recognize the limits of your professional competence.
- Be honest and trustworthy.
- Respect and protect confidential information.
- Make sure that your personal beliefs do not prejudice your patients' care.
- Act quickly to protect patients from risk if you have good reason to believe that you or a colleague may not be fit to practise.
- Avoid abusing your position as a doctor.
- Work with colleagues in the ways that best serve patients' interests.
In all these matters you must never discriminate unfairly against your patients or colleagues. And you must always be prepared to justify your actions to them.'

GMC 'Good Medical Practice' 2001 and 'Tomorrow's Doctors'

In August 2001 the GMC set out the standards of knowledge, skills and behaviour required by registered practitioners in the latest edition of its publication 'Good Medical Practice'.

'Tomorrow's Doctors' was first published in 1993, and a new edition was published in July 2002. It set out a new approach to undergraduate education, which focused on equipping students with the necessary knowledge, skills and attributes to work effectively and to continue learning and adapting to changing circumstances during their professional lives. The new edition stresses the legal and ethical basis of medicine, multi-professional working and the preparation of students to work in a multicultural society.

Standards in medical education and pre-registration training

The Education Committee is one of the statutory committees of the GMC, with a responsibility to ensure medical standards in education and in the pre-registration year for house officers. This function is fulfilled by inspections and by the monitoring of those bodies awarding qualifications and providing training. If standards of education or training were to prove inadequate the GMC might decide that the qualifications offered should no longer be recognized.

Maintaining the medical register

Doctors may be accorded provisional, limited or full registration by the GMC. Within the next few years all doctors will be required to undergo revalidation every 5 years to maintain the full privileges of registration.

Provisional registration enables the doctor to act as a registered practitioner under supervision at an approved hospital.

For limited registration a doctor must have a recognized medical qualification and have been accepted for employment in a hospital in the UK or Isle of Man. The Registrar also needs to be satisfied that the doctor has an acceptable standard of English, is of good character and has the necessary skill, knowledge and experience (Medical Act 1983, s. 22). Limited registration is for 5 years, and allows the doctor to practise under supervision and in a limited capacity.

The council for the regulation of health care professionals

Under the 2002 Act the Council for the Regulation of Health Care Professionals can investigate and report on the performance of a regulatory body such as the GMC and make recommendations as to how it performs its functions. The Council may not intervene in the actual determination of a 'fitness to practise' case, but it may refer the case to the High Court (or the Court of Session in Scotland) if it is felt that this would be desirable for the protection of members of the public. However, it is envisaged that this would only occur in extreme cases where there is a public interest in having what is regarded as a perverse decision reviewed by the High Court. It would then be for the court, not the Council, to substitute its own decision or to refer the case back to the regulatory body for a re-hearing.

The 2002 Act removes the right of doctors to appeal to the Judicial Committee of the Privy Council, and redirects appeals from doctors and dentists to the High Court.

Conclusion*

There are now a number of procedures in place to regulate professional conduct and medical practice at both an individual and an organizational level. NHS complaints procedures investigate individual complaints about patient care and are aimed at identifying and rectifying fault, and not at providing compensation. Clinical governance, risk management and audit may help to reduce medical mishaps at an organizational level, while NICE, CHAI, NSFs and the National Patient Safety Agency and Patients' Forums set out standards of care that can be expected by patients. Annual appraisal and revalidation aim to improve professional performance through peer review, promoting continuing professional development and ensuring that registered medical practitioners remain clinically competent. Alongside these measures there remain disciplinary procedures for both hospital doctors and general practitioners, who can still be held to account through the GMC and the courts.

Medical mishaps are a fact of clinical practice. There are clearly a large number of mechanisms in place to reduce adverse clinical events. It remains to be seen if the right balance will be achieved in practice between the educational and the punitive models of professional regulation.

Keypoints

- Medical mishaps are inevitable in clinical practice and have considerable human and economic costs.
- It is important to be aware of the range of professional and legal procedures in place to regulate clinical practice at both individual and organizational levels.
- Complaints procedures aim to reduce clinical adverse events by a combination of better education and disciplinary measures.

Chapter 15

Presenting evidence and rules of procedure

Learning objectives

Practical application
- How to respond to a complaint
- How to prepare a witness statement
- How to give evidence

Introduction

Complaints are an everyday fact of life for medical practitioners. We feel that it is useful to say something of complaints and how to handle them. They may cause a great deal of upset to all concerned, and may be very time-consuming. This chapter is aimed at showing some of the practicalities involved in handling complaints.

There will be times in most medical careers when doctors will be required to give evidence either as an expert witness, a witness of fact or a defendant in cases of clinical negligence. Medical practitioners may be required to appear before Independent Reviews, the General Medical Council, a Coroner, or a court in civil, or less commonly, in criminal proceedings. A court appearance may be a harrowing experience for which doctors have very little training or preparation. The purpose of this chapter is to offer some practical help and advice both in preparing reports and in explaining court procedures.

Preparing evidence (Table 15.1)

- Medical reports may be required as part of general witness statements, reports to Coroners, NHS Trust legal departments, hospital enquiries and independent reviews. For criminal and civil proceedings separate advice should be sought from solicitors.
- Statements should be headed 'Confidential' and addressed specifically to the individual, office or court requesting the report. Correspondence and communications with solicitors are usually covered by legal professional privilege, but should nevertheless be labelled 'without prejudice' in the heading.
- It is useful to begin a report with a heading followed by a short biography with your qualifications and a statement as to why you are writing the report. It is useful here to indicate the source of your information, e.g. personal knowledge and recollection of the patient, medical records, radiological and laboratory results, or post mortem findings.
- You should indicate how you encountered the patient with the relevant background information. There then follows a chronological statement, concentrating on the facts and the writer's involvement in the case. Explicit or implicit criticism of colleagues should be avoided wherever possible.
- Statements should be written in plain English, avoiding medical jargon and using short sen-

Table 15.1 Outline scheme for a witness statement or medical report

CONFIDENTIAL	For example in medical reports, which should always be marked confidential
WITHOUT PREJUDICE	Correspondence between solicitors and clients is subject to legal professional privilege; but nevertheless this should be added to the heading.
IN THE MATTER OF . . .	Reason for statement, e.g. court cases
MEDICAL REPORT ON . . .	Medical report, e.g. in an insurance claim
WITNESS STATEMENT	**Begin thus:** **I [NAME/PROFESSIONAL ADDRESS] say as follows,** name of witness/expert witness/referee (court cases only)
BIOGRAPHY AND QUALIFICATIONS	Useful where the witness is an expert witness or if it is necessary to indicate the professional reason for the involvement of the witness in the case e.g. casualty officer, pathologist
SOURCES OF INFORMATION	For example, personal observations, hospital notes, post mortem findings, etc.
STATEMENT	Usually given in numbered paragraphs for easy reference in court cases. Headings may be useful.
OPINION	It is important for expert medical referees to express their opinion in the statement and to highlight the opinion paragraph accordingly.
STATEMENT OF TRUTH	**To the best of my knowledge and belief the facts stated in this witness statement are true.** Typical phraseology in court cases only; the witness statement should conclude with this statement, clearly marked 'Statement of Truth'.
DATE AT END	**Signed . . .** **NAME OF WITNESS** **Date . . .**

tences. Paragraphs may be numbered. The report should be signed and dated and a copy should be kept. Legal advice may need to be obtained if you have concerns about potential criticism that may be directed towards you, or others. A request for your fee may be sent in a separate covering letter.

Written responses to complaints

Most complaints will require a written response. The following advice may be helpful in composing a reply to a patient's or relative's criticism.
- Reply promptly—many complaints are aggravated by delayed responses or, worse, by being ignored altogether.
- Identify precisely the complaint and respond to it.
- In order to try and resolve rather than aggravate the complaint, be courteous, objective and professional.
- Clarify the facts before responding. This may require obtaining the notes and comments or reports from others.
- Be aware of the need for confidentiality, particularly when the complainant is not the patient.
- Do not be afraid of apologizing or offering condolences, as appropriate. To express sorrow at the course of events and offer sympathy is not the same as admitting liability. However, be careful not to make any admissions of liability.
- Avoid blaming others, however strong the temptation to exonerate yourself at their expense. Beware of turning yourself into a hostile witness against your colleagues.
- Write a clear statement devoid of jargon that can be easily understood. Include information on what the claimant can do if unsatisfied with the response given—if this has not already been given by the Complaints Manager
- Get advice from the Trust solicitors, if necessary, and ask them to check the letter before it is sent.
In cases handled by others, such as the Complaints Manager or CEO, ask to see the final submission and the outcome of the complaint.

Conciliation

Conciliation is a means of complaint resolution that is usually employed when in-house procedures have not proved satisfactory to the complainant. However, some complaints managers now use conciliation in parallel with the formal hospital complaints procedures.

Conciliation is tailored to the circumstances of the individual complaint. Hence there is no set process that is adopted. Often, however, the complainant will wish a friend or some independent person to attend and provide support. Meetings between aggrieved patients and healthcare professionals can be stressful for all concerned, but do provide time and opportunity for issues to be aired, misunderstandings settled and apologies offered. Saying sorry is not an admission of legal liability; but care should be taken when doing so not to admit liability. Conciliation is essentially a private matter between the complainant and healthcare professionals. If the complaint goes to independent review, what has been said in conciliation should remain confidential.

This needs to be made clear at the start of the conciliation appointment, and all discussions to be treated as 'without prejudice', meaning that they are meant to be an attempt to reach a settlement, and thus anything said cannot later be put before a court in evidence. The courts are at pains to persuade parties to litigation to settle out of court, and settlements would be made very difficult if concessions made in the course of negotiations could thereafter be put to the court in evidence.

Giving oral evidence in court

In Coroner's, civil and criminal courts, evidence is given on oath or after affirmation. This is the point after which false evidence may be regarded as perjury. A witness should provide evidence that is:
- Factual—avoid opinions, guesses and speculation.
- Accurate—refer to notes as necessary.
- Relevant—keep answers brief and focused.
- If you do not know the answer then say so.

Some practical tips in giving evidence

- Familiarize yourself with the necessary facts of the case. Know where you can find the relevant information in the notes. You will not want to be caught out by not knowing the results of investigations or findings at operation or post mortem.
- Take your time. A conscientious witness will take sufficient time to give a truthful and accurate answer. If necessary, refer to your notes.
- If you do not understand the question, ask for clarification before you answer.
- Address the Judge/Coroner/Chairman, as he is the court to whom you are giving evidence. Observing the judge's pen will ensure that he is not having difficulty keeping up with your evidence and obviate any need to repeat it. It will also mean that you are less distracted by the questioning barrister.
- Do not 'fence' with lawyers. Their job is to ask questions on behalf of their client. Yours is to provide factual evidence for the court. The best witnesses remain calm and neutral, with no axe to grind.
- As a general rule, keep answers short. Supplementary questions can be asked if more detail or clarification is required.

Witnesses of fact will be largely confined to factual evidence. Expert witnesses, e.g. forensic pathologists, may also be asked their opinion as to the meaning or significance of the facts. Expert witnesses may be called upon to advise the court on the standard of medical care given and the probable consequences of failures in medical management.

Civil proceedings

Introduction

Civil proceedings is the term given to the rules and procedures of the civil courts. Most clinical negligence claims are civil actions.

In July 1996 Lord Woolf (the Master of the Rolls, the senior judge of the Court of Appeal for civil cases), published a report called 'Access to Justice', on changes to the civil justice system. The main recommendations were incorporated into new Civil Procedure Rules (CPR), which replace the old Rules of the Supreme Court. The principles behind the new rules, which now govern civil litigation, are:

- Litigation should be a measure of last resort.
- Alternative dispute resolution (ADR) is to be encouraged.
- There should be improved case management, with judges acting as trial managers with powers to set timetables, cap costs and impose sanctions.
- There will now be three trial tracks:
  —a small-claims track for disputes valued up to £5,000 damages.
  —a fast-track system for disputes lasting no more than one day in court.
  —a multi-track system for more complex cases.
- There will now be a single set of rules for all civil courts.
- There will now be improved access to information technology.

Civil procedure rules

The new Civil Procedure Rules now govern the way clinical negligence is conducted, with greater emphasis on out-of-court settlements, the use of alternative dispute resolution and conciliation, management of cases by judges, use of expert witnesses and pre-trial conferences to clarify the issues before the courts.

The emphasis upon settlement rather than litigation can result in more pre-trial activity and surprisingly swift settlements at court when, seemingly, the case has hardly begun. This can be difficult for the layman to understand; but there are now strong pressures on litigants to avoid the costs of litigation, and hence such settlements often occur at the door of the court or mid-way through trial.

Case management

The court now has greater flexibility in the management of a case. It will seek to tailor its directions to the needs of the situation and the steps the parties have taken to prepare the case. It will be concerned with ensuring that the issues are properly identified and the necessary evidence is prepared and disclosed early on.

Hence, the court may intervene regarding:
- The timing of a trial date
- Case Management conferences
- Disclosure of documents
- Provision of factual and expert evidence
- Use of single experts
- Exchange of expert evidence and 'without prejudice' discussions between experts
- Pre-trial reviews.

Case Management Conferences

At a Case Management Conference (CMC) the court will review the steps taken by the parties to prepare the case, give any directions to help progress the claim and to ensure, if possible, that the parties agree the matters at issue. The parties and their legal advisers should ensure that the necessary documentation (including witness statements and expert reports) is available for the CMC. Legal authority or references may be used to assist the court to understand and deal with the questions before it, and it may be necessary to include a brief chronological account of the claim, the facts that are agreed, and those that are in dispute, and of the evidence that is needed to decide them. A case summary should be prepared by the claimant and be agreed with the other parties, if possible.

Topics that the court will usually consider will include:
- whether the claimant has made clear what he is claiming and the amount claimed
- any amendments to the claim
- the disclosure of documents
- what factual evidence should be disclosed
- what expert evidence is required
- the need for clarification of issues and questions to be put to the experts.

A direction giving permission to use expert evidence will indicate whether this will be in the form of oral or written evidence and will name the experts concerned. A CMC may also consider whether the case should be tried by a High Court judge or a judge specializing in that particular type of claim. Sanctions may be imposed for failure to comply with directions given by the court at a CMC, and these are typically by making a party pay the costs of the time wasted. This is an effective penalty, since costs may be expensive.

Pre-trial checklist

A pre-trial checklist (Civil Court Form N170, available from the Court Service website) is issued not later than 8 weeks before the trial and placed before the judge for his directions. The court may also decide to hold a pre-trial review (PTR).

The trial

Clinical negligence cases are usually held without a jury. The trial judge will normally have read the papers in the trial bundle, and may dispense with an opening address by Counsel. The court has power (CPR rule 32.1) to control the evidence and restrict cross-examination, and under CPR rule 32.5(2) to determine the statements and reports that are to stand as evidence in chief. Most witness statements will normally stand as evidence in chief without the need for the witness to give his evidence orally. Cross-examination follows directly after. This saves time and thus costs, but does mean that witness statements must be thoroughly prepared. Once the trial has begun, the judge will normally sit on consecutive days until it is concluded.

Conclusion

The Woolf recommendations have largely been implemented in practice. Clinical negligence claims are stressful, and often long-drawn-out and expensive. The Woolf Recommendations and the new Civil Procedure Rules emphasize the importance of alternative dispute resolution (ADR), and the courts may enquire of the parties the extent to which these have been used. Clearly, in the case of clinical negligence cases, there are a number of means of resolving disputes through the hospital complaints procedures and independent reviews outlined in Chapter 14. The courts may well expect these to be used. As Lord Woolf pointed out, litigation should be a means of last resort.

However, when cases do proceed to litigation, the new Civil Procedure Rules seek to clarify the issues, control the use of evidence, including medical expert statements, shorten the time to completion and reduce costs. The conduct of the case will be more directly under the control of the court than was the case before the new rules came into force. In clinical negligence cases, much is decided by the medical evidence and the expert witnesses. The primary duty of the expert witness is to the court, not to any particular party. Case Management Conferences and meetings of experts aim to clarify the points at issue and determine what is agreed and what is in dispute before the trial takes place. Again, this saves time and costs, which is in the interests of all parties.

Glossary of terms used in civil litigation

Affidavit	A written, sworn statement of evidence
Alternative dispute resolution (ADR)	Collective description of methods used to resolve disputes otherwise than through the normal trial process
Counterclaim	A claim brought by the defendant in response to the claimant's claim
Cross examination	Questioning of a witness, including an expert witness, by a party other than the party who called the witness
Damages	A sum of money awarded by the court to the claimant as compensation
Aggravated damages	Additional damages awarded as compensation for the defendant's objectionable behaviour
Exemplary damages	Damages that go beyond compensation for actual loss, which are awarded to show the court's disapproval of the defendant's behaviour, usually where the defendant is a public authority that has exceeded its constitutional rights
Evidence in chief	The evidence given by a witness for the party who called him
Indemnity	A right of someone to recover from a third party the whole amount that he is liable to pay. For example, NHS doctors are covered by an NHS Indemnity Scheme for clinical negligence.
Injunction	A court order prohibiting a person from doing something, or requiring a person to do something
Joint liability	All those who are jointly liable share a single liability and each party can be held liable for the whole of it. For example, doctors working in a multidisciplinary team may share joint liability for a clinically adverse event.
Limitation period	The period during which a person has a right to claim against another person and must start court proceedings. The expiration of this period may be a defence to a claim.
Practice form	A form to be used for a particular purpose in proceedings according to a practice direction
Pre-action protocol	Statements of understanding between legal practitioners and others about pre-trial practice that are covered by the relevant practice direction in the Civil Procedure Rules. They are designed to ensure that avenues of ADR have been explored before litigation commences.
Privilege	The right of a party to refuse to disclose or produce a document or refuse to answer questions on the ground of some special interest recognized by law.
Several liability	A person who is severally liable with others may remain liable for the whole claim even where judgment has been obtained against the others.
Without prejudice	Negotiations with a view to settlement are usually conducted without prejudice, which means that the circumstances in which the content of the negotiations may be revealed to the court are limited.

Chapter 16

The Coroner's court

It is likely that most doctors in the acute specialities will present evidence to the Coroner (or Procurator Fiscal in Scotland). Most doctors will sign death certificates and will need to know when to refer cases to the Coroner's officer. Some explanation of the procedures of the Coroner's court and the possible decisions that can be reached is important. Many doctors and nurses fail to understand that while the Coroner's court has a judicial function, it is not there to apportion blame to specific individuals. However, the Procurator in Scotland, unlike his English counterpart, may also act as a prosecuting officer.

Coroner's court

The office of Coroner is over eight hundred years old, and is a uniquely English Institution. Scotland never adopted a Coronial system. (For a brief history of the office of Coroner see Box 16.1.)

It is likely that most clinicians will at some stage be required to attend a Coroner's Inquest. Attendance is a legal requirement if requested by the Coroner. However, a well-written medical report may obviate the need for oral evidence. The purpose of an Inquest is to establish the cause of death, not to apportion blame to particular individuals (Table 16.1). Indeed, the Coroners' Rules specifically forbid identifying any individuals by name who may have criminal or civil liability for the death.

Reporting deaths to the Coroner

The Coroner is an independent judicial officer empowered to enquire into the circumstances surrounding deaths to establish when, where and how the deceased came to his or her death.

The Coroner (or Procurator Fiscal in Scotland) should be notified in cases of sudden death, if the cause of death is unknown or there is any suggestion that the death arose from medical error or accident or was the result of industrial disease (Table 16.2). Relatives of the deceased may also contact the Coroner if they are concerned about the circumstances surrounding the death. In Scotland, this is a common practice, particularly if there is a suspicion of clinical negligence. Unlike the English Coroner, the Procurator Fiscal may also act as a prosecutor.

Box 16.1 A brief history of the office of Coroner

Historically the most important role of the Coroner was the investigation of sudden death, which survives to the present day. Murder, manslaughter, accidental and natural deaths and suicides all came to the attention of the Coroner. Failure to inform the Coroner of a death was a serious offence, and the offending township would suffer heavily for it. Those discovering a murder victim would have to raise the 'hue and cry' and initiate the hunt for the killer. Failure to preserve the body for the Coroner to view was also illegal, and punishable by substantial fines payable to the King. The Coroner's obligation to inspect the corpse continued up until 1980. The Coroner had a duty to view the body to detect any sign of violence and then to hold an inquest. It was only in 1836 that the Coroner was allowed to pay a medical witness to assist at post mortem examinations. Medieval inquests required juries consisting entirely of males of over twelve years from the nearest townships. These jurors were hence also potential witnesses.

The Coroner also had other duties, such as examining women after rape and the victims of non-fatal woundings (almost like a modern police surgeon). In the case of a non-fatal wounding, the accused would not face arrest or imprisonment before trial, but had to find four people to stand surety for him and put up 'bail money'. This was carefully recorded by the Coroner, who would arrange for the forfeiture of the bail money if the miscreant absconded.

A further duty of the Coroner, which is contained in a statute of Edward I in 1275 and persists to this day, is in relation to treasure trove. Before banks, wealth could only be concealed on the person or in hiding-places. Any such rediscovered buried treasure was of major importance as a source of Crown revenue. Further odd responsibilities of Coroners, again linked to the financial considerations of the Crown, were in relation to 'wrecks of the sea' and the investigation of catches of royal fish — the whale and the sturgeon. These duties in relation to wrecks and royal fish were only abolished by the Coroners Act of 1887.

Table 16.1 Purpose of a Coroner's Inquest

According to Rule 36 of the Coroners' Rules 1984:

• The proceedings and evidence at an inquest shall be directed solely to ascertaining the following matters, namely
    • who the deceased was;
    • how, when and where the deceased came by his death;
    • the particulars for the time being required by the Registration Act to be registered concerning the death.
 • Neither the coroner nor the jury shall express any opinion on any other matters.

Table 16.2 Cases that a doctor should refer to the Coroner

A doctor should notify the Coroner in cases:
• of sudden death of unknown cause;   • where a clinical adverse event or accident is suspected;   • of industrial disease;   • where relatives are concerned about the circumstances of a death, e.g. in cases of foul play, medical negligence, accident or neglect;   • where the death occurred in prison or a young offender's institution (there is no duty to report deaths of patients compulsorily detained in a mental hospital, which are provided for under other laws.)

It is an offence to bury or cremate a body in order to prevent investigation by the Coroner or to obstruct the Coroner in the exercise of his duty.

There is no statutory obligation for any doctor to notify a death to the Coroner. The law is satisfied if he issues a death certificate, and it is then left to the Registrar of Births and Deaths to inform the Coroner. The Registrar of Deaths has a statutory obligation to notify the Coroner in the following circumstances:

• Where the deceased was not seen by a doctor after death or within 14 days prior to death.

• Where the deceased was not attended by a registered practitioner during the last illness.

• In case of deaths occurring during surgery or within 24 hours of the operation or full recovery from the anaesthetic or where the death is thought to be related to the surgery or the anaesthetic.

• Where the Registrar cannot complete the certificate of cause of death, or where the cause of death is unknown.

• In the case of any death felt to be unnatural or caused by violence, neglect, or illegal abortion, or which is attended by suspicious circumstances.
• In the case of any death ascribed by the medical certificate to industrial disease or industrial poisoning.
• In the case of any 'stillbirth' where there is reason to believe that the child was born alive.

The Registrar will not be able to register a death until permission has been granted by the Coroner.

Before the inquest

Coroners are independent judicial officers. This means that no one else can direct them or tell them what they should do. Nevertheless, they must follow the laws and regulations that apply to their duties. The principal legislation governing their statutory duties is the Coroners Act 1988 and the Coroners Rules 1985. Coroners' decisions are subject to judicial review by the High court.

Coroners have a statutory duty to investigate deaths reported to them except where the cause of sudden or unnatural death is the subject of criminal proceedings. Inquests are also held if a person dies in prison or (usually) whenever someone dies in police custody. Reasons for referring deaths to the Coroner are listed in Table 16.1. Where a person is charged with homicide, the inquest on the victim must be adjourned at the request of the chief officer of police. The case is then referred to the Crown Prosecution Service for investigation and criminal proceedings. The inquest may be resumed after the trial at the discretion of the Coroner. However, if the inquest is resumed, its findings must be consistent with the outcome of the criminal trial. Only a small number (currently 12%) of deaths reported to the Coroner will result in an inquest. After considering the evidence the Coroner may decide that an inquest is unnecessary, whereupon a death certificate is sent to the Registrar of deaths within 5 days of the completion of the Coroner's enquiries. Where preliminary interviews are required by the Coroner or his staff, they should be conducted at a time and place convenient to the person concerned, avoiding any additional distress.

Post mortem examinations

When the Coroner decides that a post mortem is required, the next of kin are entitled to an explanation and notice of the arrangements (where practicable), so that they may be represented by a medical practitioner if they so wish. Unfortunately, few members of the public are aware of this right. It is common, in cases of disputed findings, for the family solicitor to commission a second post mortem. Most Coroners will comply with such a request, but it is unclear whether they are legally obliged to. A copy of the post mortem report may be sent to interested parties on request and at the Coroner's discretion.

Juries

Some inquests involve jurors, who will also be notified of their duties and be given an indication of how long the jury service will last. Juries are required where there is reason to suspect that the death occurred:
• in prison
• as a result of an industrial accident, poisoning or disease, notice of which is required to be given
• in police custody or as a result of injury caused by a police officer
• in circumstances the continuance or possible recurrence of which is prejudicial to the health or safety of the public or any section of the public.

The Coroner has discretion in other cases. Coroners' juries have between seven and eleven members, who are summoned from the electoral roll.

The inquest proceedings: formal opening

This is usually a brief hearing at the Coroner's court to hear formal evidence about the identity of the person and for the Coroner to sign a form allowing burial or cremation of the body. The inquest is then adjourned, usually for several weeks, pending the full hearing.

Inquest

An inquest is a formal court hearing. It is open to the public, and the press may be present. Nevertheless, because of the disturbing nature of inquests, and to avoid distress to relatives the Coroner may direct that sensitive material, such as suicide notes, is not read out in court.

The deceased is first formally identified, and statements may be taken from members of the family at the discretion of the Coroner. Witnesses are then called, and the post-mortem findings are given by the pathologist. Witnesses must be either sworn or give an affirmation. Medical witnesses will be expected to have the necessary documentation to hand, e.g. medical notes.

Involvement of interested persons

Any 'properly interested persons' have a right to question witnesses either in person or through a barrister or solicitor. However, unlike other legal hearings, legal aid/public funding is not available to those wishing to be represented at an inquest. The 'interested persons' include the family and anyone who has some connection with the deceased or the events leading up to the death. It is the duty of the Coroner to call witnesses. However, important witnesses may be overlooked, and interested persons may write to the Coroner indicating whom they may wish to question through their lawyer. Only questions regarded as 'relevant' and 'proper' by the Coroner may be put to witnesses. Legal representatives are not permitted to summarize or interpret the evidence, as is done in criminal or civil proceedings.

The verdict

The conclusion reached by the Coroner or jury should be solely based on the evidence given at the inquest. Nevertheless, preliminary inquiries by the police or Coroner's officer (usually a police officer) may already point to a particular conclusion, and this may be reflected in the conduct of the inquest.

An inquest does not decide questions of civil or criminal liability. Any verdict that appears to deter-

mine the criminal liability or civil liability of a named person is forbidden. Nevertheless, the Coroner may bring a verdict of 'unlawful killing' as long as the killer is not named, or of 'lack of care' while not legally implying civil liability.

The commonest verdicts are:
- natural causes
- accident
- misadventure
- suicide
- an open verdict.

Suicide and unlawful killing require proof 'beyond reasonable doubt', as in criminal trials, while the other verdicts can be arrived at 'on the balance of probabilities'. The Coroner has no power to commit anyone for trial for an offence. Coroners are still permitted to make recommendations to prevent further deaths. However, juries can no longer add 'riders' to their verdict. An open verdict is given when there is insufficient information to point to a definite cause of death, e.g. when the deceased may have brought about their own death, but it is not clear whether they intended to do so, as in the case of an elderly person living alone with severe coronary artery disease who is found dead having ingested a large number of sleeping tablets.

Appeals against the verdict

There is no appeal from the decision of an inquest, although the verdict may be overturned if the Coroner has made an error of law or if significant new evidence comes to light. Errors of law can be challenged by applying to the Divisional court for judicial review within three months (but preferably earlier). Alternatively, an application can be made to the Attorney General for a 'fiat', which, if allowed, permits application to the Divisional court. The Divisional court will only overturn a verdict if it would have been different had the inquest been conducted correctly or new evidence had been known. If the verdict is overturned, another inquest is usually held by another Coroner.

After the inquest

The next of kin will be provided with an explana-

Table 16.3 Steps in a Coroner's Inquiry

Deaths to be reported to the Coroner by the Registrar
• Where deceased not seen by a doctor within 14 days or during last illness
• Where Registrar cannot complete death certificate
• Deaths—within 24 hours of surgery or general anaesthetic, or thought to be due to:
• unnatural causes,
• violence,
• neglect,
• suspicious circumstances,
• illegal abortion,
• industrial disease
• industrial poisoning
• alleged stillbirth where the child may have been born alive.
Before the Inquest
• Next of kin informed of arrangements of post mortem and inquest. Relatives may be represented by
• a doctor
• a solicitor.
• Selection of a jury where appropriate
Formal opening of Inquest
• Identification of deceased
• Grant permission for burial or cremation
• Adjournment for formal inquest
Full hearing
• Statements from family and relatives (at discretion of Coroner)
• Witness Statements, including Pathologist's report of post-mortem
• Coroner may allow 'proper and relevant' questions from interested parties
Verdict
• Reached by Coroner or Jury.
• Cannot determine civil or criminal liability.
• Cases of unlawful killing or death through neglect must not identify suspect(s).
After the Inquest
• Death certificate issued.
• Coroner may issue a report to the relevant persons or authority to prevent further deaths.

tion of how, where and when a copy of the death certificate may be obtained. If, in the interests of preventing further deaths, the Coroner decides to report the matter to the relevant person or authority, he will also send a copy of his letter to all inter-

ested parties. Complaints about a Coroner's decision can only be made and the result of an inquest can only be challenged through the High court.

The Procurator Fiscal Service in Scotland

The Crown Office and Procurator Fiscal Service constitutes the sole public prosecuting authority in Scotland and forms part of the Scottish Executive. It is led by the Lord Advocate, whose authority in relation to criminal prosecution and the investigation of deaths in Scotland is enshrined in the Scotland Act 1998. The Procurators Fiscal are qualified lawyers and permanent civil servants who hold commissions from the Lord Advocate. The Procurator has wide-ranging powers in relation to the investigation of crime, including complaints of criminal conduct by police officers, supervision of charities and the administration of property falling into *bona vacantia* (ownerless property that passes to the Crown) or treasure trove.

The Procurator Fiscal is empowered to investigate all sudden deaths and, where appropriate, conduct public enquiries. In this respect, the functions of the Procurator Fiscal extend beyond those of the Coroner, since the Procurator, unlike his English and Welsh counterparts, has responsibility for the investigation and prosecution of crime in the public interest, as well as for the investigation of sudden, suspicious or unexplained deaths and for conducting Fatal Accident Inquiries. They investigate round 14,000 sudden deaths per year. Fatal Accident Inquiries (FAIs) are required for certain categories of death, such as those occurring in custody. The Lord Advocate has discretion in holding FAIs in other cases.

Differences between the Coroner and Procurator Fiscal (Table 16.4)

The Procurator, unlike the Coroner, may act as a prosecutor, and is always legally qualified. His main role is to determine whether death has arisen from crime or neglect. The Procurator is therefore not obliged to investigate the precise cause of death once it is established that it is due to natural

Table 16.4 Differences between the roles of Coroner and Procurator Fiscal

Coroner System	Procurator Fiscal System
Coroners are legally or medically qualified and often part-time.	Procurators are full-time legally qualified civil servants.
Responsible to Lord Chancellor.	Responsible to Lord Advocate.
Inquests held in public.	Proceedings not always public.
	Procurator has powers of precognition.
	Procurator usually presides over confidential inquiries into sudden or unexpected deaths.
Inquests may be held with a Jury.	Fatal Accident Inquiries held by Sheriff without a Jury.
Coroner's post mortems usually performed by single pathologist.	Post mortems for deaths due to drugs or subject to criminal proceedings performed by two doctors.
Limited range of verdicts.	Wide range of verdicts made by determination.
Determines circumstances and cause of death only.	Investigates circumstances and cause of death, and may instigate criminal proceedings.
Cannot apportion criminal or civil liability to identifiable individuals.	Individuals identified in Fatal Accident Inquiries, which are held in Sheriff court.
Inquests are adjourned during criminal proceedings.	
Coroner does not usually deal directly with members of the public before inquest.	Procurator may discuss cases with relatives, especially where there may be a medical mishap.

causes. As in England and Wales, the Registrar of Births and Deaths is the only person with a legal obligation to inform the Procurator. However, it is recommended that a doctor inform the Procurator whenever there is doubt about the cause or circumstances of a death. In contrast to the situation in England and Wales, relatives of the deceased may approach the Procurator directly where they are

concerned about the circumstances of a death that may have arisen from a medical mishap. Rule 12 of the Crown Office publication, *Death and the Procurator Fiscal*, states that the Procurator should be informed of:

'any death as a result of a medical mishap, and any death where a complaint is received which suggests that medical treatment or the absence of treatment may have contributed to the death'.

There is no '24 hour rule' for deaths related to surgery or anaesthetics, as in England and Wales.

A form F89 should be completed and sent to the Procurator, giving the details of the medical care and death. The police may or may not be involved. The issues of interest to the procurator are whether:
• the patient was adequately examined by the doctors;
• all due precautions were taken in the medical management, including the use of diagnostic procedures, anaesthetics and medication;
• any factors could or should have been known that would indicate that the medical management would be attended by any special risk to life.

The Procurator may examine witnesses by precognition, which is a private interrogation aimed at clarifying or amplifying the preliminary statements of witnesses. If the Procurator is then satisfied that there is no criminality or negligence involved in a sudden death, he may decide not to pursue matters on his own responsibility. However, as in England and Wales, there are certain categories of death that require him to report the circumstances to the Crown Office.

Such deaths include those:
• that have occurred under suspicious circumstances
• where criminal proceedings may be instituted
• where a Public Inquiry has been, or will be, held
• involving possible suicide
• involving medical mishap, or abuse of volatile substances
• occurring as an accident in the course of voluntary or charitable work
• where there might be future risk to public health and safety

- of members of the armed forces or police in the course of their duties
- involving fire or explosion
- where the Procurator is of the opinion the death ought to be referred.

A Public Inquiry may be requested by an appropriate interested party (usually relatives), and may be held where the Procurator Fiscal deems it appropriate under the Fatal Accident and Sudden Deaths Inquiry (Scotland) Act 1976 or where it appears to the Lord Advocate to be expedient in the public interest.

In contrast to England, where inquests are public, in Scotland, Fatal Accident Inquiries are focused more on those deaths likely to be of public concern—including those arising from medical negligence.

At a Fatal Accident Inquiry the Sheriff sits without a jury. Witnesses cannot be compelled to answer questions that would indicate that they are guilty of a crime or offence.

The Sheriff then determines:
- when, where and how the death(s) took place;
- the cause of death and any precautions that might have prevented it;
- any other relevant facts e.g. organizational failures contributing to the death.

Unlike the Coroner, the Sheriff in a Fatal Accident Inquiry does not have a choice of verdicts, but simply makes a determination as to the cause of death.

Differences between the role of the Coroner and Procurator are summarized in Table 16.4.

Chapter 17

The General Medical Council

Learning objectives

Core knowledge
- Statutory functions and powers of the GMC
- When the GMC may take action

Practical applications
- Know when to seek help and advice from the GMC

Background principles
- Importance of maintaining good medical practice
- Need to protect the public
- Differences between poor performance and underperformance and professional misconduct

The General Medical Council

The General Medical Council (GMC) licenses doctors to practise and has a statutory duty to foster good medical practice, promote high standards of training, and—deal firmly and fairly with those doctors whose fitness to practise is in doubt (Table 17.1).

In 1980 health procedures were introduced that meant that the GMC could investigate doctors whose performance was adversely affected by ill-health. Hitherto the GMC could only have taken action in cases of doctors with serious health problems if they committed a crime or were engaged in serious professional misconduct. In 1997 the GMC introduced performance procedures that enabled it to tackle seriously deficient performance by re-quiring doctors to undergo retraining. Both the health and the performance procedures emphasized remedial action rather than punishment, although doctors can be removed from practice in the interests of patient welfare.

Table 17.2 lists matters not usually coming within the remit of the GMC.

Causes for action by the GMC

The GMC may take action against a doctor:
- Who has been convicted of a criminal offence in a British court.
- When there is an allegation of serious professional misconduct.
- When the doctor's professional performance is regarded as seriously deficient.
- When the doctor is attempting to practise when physically or mentally unfit.

The central issue in all these cases is whether the doctor remains fit to practise as judged by the standards of clinical practice and ethics set out in *Good Medical Practice*. As always, the safety of the public is of paramount importance.

Sources of referral to the GMC

In 1998 of the 190,000 doctors registered with the GMC, there were 2,863 complaints (against 1.5% of doctors), as a result of which action was taken against 620 doctors and 22 were struck off. Hence,

Table 17.1 Statutory functions of the GMC

The GMC has four main functions recognized in law: ● Keeping an up-to-date register of qualified doctors ● Fostering good medical practice ● Promoting high standards of medical education ● Dealing firmly but fairly with doctors whose fitness to practise is in doubt.

Table 17.2 Matters outside the powers of the GMC

The GMC will *not* normally become involved with: ● Minor cases and occasional poor performance ● The doctor's contract, where it is not relevant to registration ● Performance targets set by management ● Behaviour that does not affect the doctor's professional work or position, except where it has led to a criminal conviction. *Maintaining Good Medical Practice* (GMC 2001)

in the majority of cases (2,243) no action was taken. The reasons included:

● frivolous complaints;
● insufficient evidence;
● anonymous accusations; and
● the fact that the complaint was about health services not involving doctors or had no bearing on the doctor's fitness to practise.

In 2000 the number of complaints to the GMC had risen to 4,470 (2.3% of doctors).

Complaints come mainly from two sources:

● following convictions for criminal offences; or
● as allegations from individuals or organizations.

The police have standing instructions to refer those with criminal convictions to the GMC. Since the GMC must accept the convictions of British courts, it is important that doctors do not plead guilty to crime unless guilty. The preliminary proceedings committee will normally be interested in those convictions bearing on fitness to practise, and will not normally consider:

● minor motoring convictions;
● convictions suggesting that the doctor has a serious health problem (which are referred to health screeners);
● convictions incurred more than 5 years previously; and

● minor convictions that would not affect medical practice or bring the profession into disrepute.

Complaints may also come from individuals such as patients and their relatives, or colleagues. The GMC hears such complaints in the form of sworn statements known as statutory declarations. Information may also come from persons acting in a public capacity, such as a member of the government or a health authority. Such individuals are not required to make sworn statements.

Initial screening

Screening may be for concerns relating to conduct, performance or health. Health screeners are medically qualified, and are often psychiatrists. Those screening for poor conduct or performance may be either medically qualified or lay persons (Figure 17.1).

Poor conduct and performance

The screener will consider whether or not the doctor might be guilty of misconduct according to the following criteria:

● the gravity of the alleged behaviour
● the number of victims
● the risk to patients and the public
● whether the doctor acted deliberately, recklessly, accidentally or in bad faith
● whether the doctor neglected his professional responsibilities
● whether the GMC had received previous complaints suggesting a pattern of behaviour amounting to serious professional misconduct.

If the screener considers that the doctor's behaviour signifies serious professional misconduct the case will be referred to the Preliminary Proceedings Committee (PPC).

If it is felt that the doctor's conduct does not warrant investigation for serious professional misconduct the screener may still consider deficiency in the doctor's performance if:

● there is evidence that since July 1997 (when these procedures began) there has been a persistent failure to achieve acceptable professional standards appropriate to his/her work;

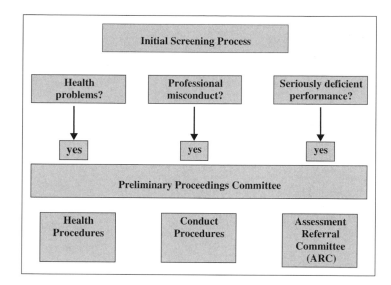

Figure 17.1. GMC Procedures.

- the evidence shows a pattern of poor performance rather than a small number of incidents that might represent isolated lapses; or
- the alleged deficiencies are so serious that, if they are not corrected, there might be grounds for restricting or suspending the doctor's registration.

The primary concern is that the doctor may be putting patients at risk and may be repeatedly and persistently failing to comply with the GMC standards as defined in *Good Medical Practice*. At this point the screener might invite comments from the doctor before deciding on whether formal assessment is required.

If the screener decides that there are no questions as to either serious professional misconduct or seriously deficient performance, the papers go to a lay screener for endorsement. If both screeners agree, the matter rests there. If the lay screener disagrees the complaint must proceed to the next stage of the conduct or performance procedures.

Where a health screener calls into question the health of a doctor, the GMC will not consider action under the conduct or performance procedures until or unless it can be established that the doctor's actions are not due to ill health.

Letters of advice

Sometimes a screener will decide that, while the case does not require further action under the fitness to practise procedures, the doctor ought to be given informal advice. With the agreement of the lay screener, the doctor will be sent a letter outlining the complaint and asking for comments or an explanation. If the screener offers advice, or a warning, the file will be kept by the GMC in case of future complaints arising.

The Professional Conduct Procedures

If the complaint goes forward the relevant papers and the doctor's comments will be forwarded to the Preliminary Proceedings Committee (PPC).

The PPC consists of seven GMC members, five medical and two non-medical. Proceedings are in private at the GMC offices. A senior lawyer is present, acting as an impartial legal assessor to advise on points of law. The press is not admitted, and the doctor is not usually called to give evidence except in unusually serious cases.

The PPC has five options:
- To take no further action.
- To defer a decision pending further information.
- To issue a warning or advice that remains on file but is not made public.
- To refer under the health or performance procedures.

- To refer for a full public hearing of the Professional Conduct Committee (PCC).

If it is decided to take the matter to the Committee on Professional Performance or the Health Committee the doctor may be suspended, or restrictions may be placed on registration, if it is in the doctor's or the public's interest, for up to 6 months. Suspension can be renewed after 3 months. However, if this is the case, the doctor can attend the PPC and be legally represented.

The Professional Conduct Committee (PCC)

A panel of the Professional Conduct Committee (PCC) consists of five members, including a non-medical member. There is a legal assessor to advise on law. The formal charges are sent to the doctor, who is advised to attend and may be legally and professionally represented, although there is no requirement for the defendant to be present.

The case against the doctor is made by the GMC's legal team. The doctor may conduct the defence, but will normally be represented by his medical defence organization, who can instruct solicitors or barristers as appropriate.

Procedure

The hearing is in public, and the press is usually present. Although the committee is not a court of law, its proceedings are similar, with evidence given on oath. Witnesses can be cross-examined by the other side and by members of the PCC panel.

Having heard the evidence the panel must decide three questions:

- Have all—or some—of the alleged facts been proved?
- Do the proved facts amount to serious professional misconduct?
- If so, what sanctions are appropriate?

The sanctions are:

- To administer an admonition in public.
- To place conditions on registration for up to three years that limit the doctor's freedom to practise. These can be renewed.

- To suspend registration for up to a year (also a renewable penalty).
- To strike off the Medical Register.

If the PCC finds the facts proved, it will hear evidence in possible mitigation before deciding on a finding of serious professional misconduct. The panel will also hear evidence relating to the doctor's previous history and character. After hearing evidence in relation to mitigating factors and character the panel will reach a verdict.

The Performance and Health Procedures

Whilst conduct procedures are adversarial and punitive in nature, performance and health procedures are, conversely, conducted along the lines of an inquiry. They aim to put right deficiencies and rehabilitate the sick doctor, while protecting the public.

Seriously deficient performance is defined by the GMC as 'a departure from good professional practice, whether or not it is covered by specific GMC guidance, sufficiently serious to call into question a doctor's registration'.

Invitation for assessment

If a GMC screener thinks that the doctor's performance may be seriously deficient he will invite the doctor for assessment before two doctors from the relevant speciality and a lay person. The doctor has 28 days to reply. If he fails to accept assessment, the case will be reviewed by the GMC's Assessment Referral Committee (ARC). The ARC may agree with the screener or drop the case. A decision for assessment by the ARC must be complied with.

The assessment

A medical member of the Council takes over as case co-ordinator. The assessment is carried out by two doctors and a lay assessor, who are not members of the GMC but have been selected and trained by the GMC following public advertisement. The team will review the case, including the doctor's comments, visit the doctor at work and interview the complainant. This investigation takes place in a low-profile way and is not publicized. The team may assess the doctor using a variety of methods, including direct observation with actual patients, testing knowledge and skills, or the use of 'standardized patients' in role play. If during the assessment the doctor decides to retire voluntarily and be removed from the register, the performance proceedings will be discontinued. However this does not normally happen with conduct proceedings, which generally run their course.

The decision following assessment

The team will report back to the case co-ordinator with their recommendation to rectify deficient performance. However, if they decide that there has not been seriously deficient performance, no further action will usually be taken. If they have identified serious deficiencies the doctor will be asked to agree to a statement of requirements to address the problems. This may include retraining, counselling or limiting practice under supervision. Such remedial action is expected to be voluntary. If the doctor fails to agree or the performance is regarded as sufficiently poor, the doctor may be referred to the Committee on Professional Performance (CPP), which will decide on suspension or placing restrictions on registration.

If the doctor agrees to rectify the deficient performance, the onus rests with him, but it remains up to the GMC to be satisfied that the standards have reached the required level. If standards do not improve, the case will be referred to the CPP.

The Committee on Professional Performance (CPP)

This Committee on Professional Performance, like the PCC, sits in panels of seven (5 medical and 2 lay members), is advised by a legal assessor on points of law, and meets in private. As with the PCC, attendance of the doctor is not required, but is advisable. Legal rules of procedure are followed, with witnesses (sometimes including the complainant) and cross-examination. The doctor is entitled to legal representation. The CPP may postpone a decision

Table 17.3 Professional Conduct Committee (PCC) and Committee on Professional Performance (CPP)

Professional Conduct Committee (PCC)	Committee on Professional Performance (CPP)
Referral	
Patients, public, doctors, courts	Patients, public, organiszations, e.g. Trusts, doctors. Self-referral.
Remit	
Serious professional misconduct	Seriously deficient performance
Penalties	
Erasure from register	
Suspend registration	Suspend registration
Place conditions on registration	Place conditions on registration
Public admonition	
Other outcomes	Voluntary retirement Counselling Training Remedial action and re-assessment
Hearing	
Public	Held in private Assessments of performance are confidential
Doctor attends hearing	Doctor well advised to attend
Appeals	
High Court	High Court
Court of Session	Court of Session
High Court of Justice (NI)	High Court of Justice (NI)

pending further evidence, suspend registration for a year, place conditions on registration for up to three years, or suspend registration indefinitely (after at least one hearing and two years' suspension). The CPP publishes findings of seriously deficient performance, and will tell enquirers about any limitations on practitioners made by the CPP.

The health procedures and the Health Committee

Impaired fitness to practise resulting from a doctor's ill health is treated entirely differently from seriously deficient performance and matters of professional or personal misconduct. Referrals can come from a variety of sources, including colleagues or even the doctor himself. The GMC reminds doctors that they are under an obligation to act if they feel that a colleague's performance is impaired through illness.

> 'You must protect patients when you believe that a colleague's conduct, performance or health is a threat to them.'
>
> *Good Medical Practice*

The case is initially taken up by a medically qualified health screener who is a member of the GMC and is often a psychiatrist. The health screener makes a preliminary inquiry and may decide that the issue can be dealt with locally without involving the GMC. It is best that health matters are dealt with early, and with as much voluntary co-operation from the doctor as possible.

The health screener may require a medical examination, usually by doctors in the local region who are not GMC members. They will report on:
- the medical condition,
- fitness to practise and the need for treatment, and
- recommendations as to how patients can be protected during the doctor's treatment or rehabilitation.

If the health screener regards the case as sufficiently serious, the doctor is informed and required to accept the appropriate remedial action. The doctor is then placed under supervision, and the supervisor is asked to report on progress to the screener. Supervision may place restrictions as to:
- the place or type of work,
- the level of responsibility,
- avoidance of stress or single-handed practice,
- abstinence from alcohol, or
- avoidance of work altogether whilst undergoing treatment.

The matters agreed are confidential, but the GMC may ask the doctor's permission to disclose information to prospective employers regarding supervision and to specify agreed limitations on clinical practice.

Provided the doctor co-operates with supervision and agrees on the recommended limitations on practice, there will be no need for a formal hearing by the GMC and there will be no formal limitations on registration. Once the screener finds that the doctor is fit to practise on the basis of the supervisor's reports, the matter is ended, unless there is recurrent illness. Nevertheless the doctor is advised to continue to seek the help and support of the supervisor and to follow their advice as long as supervisor and doctor both feel this is useful.

The Health Committee will become involved in the case if the doctor:
- refuses or fails to be examined;
- refuses to follow the recommendations of the examiners;
- fails to comply with agreed undertakings;
- suffers a deterioration in health during assessment.

The health committee consists of seven members (five are medical) and sits in private. The doctor is entitled to the same degree of confidentiality as any other patient. The committee is assisted by two medical experts. One is usually a psychiatrist (sometimes a neurologist), and the other comes from the doctor's own speciality. As with the other fitness-to-practise committees, there is also a legal assessor. The doctor is advised not to attend alone, to reduce stress, and is entitled to legal representation. While the procedures follow legal rules, they are not adversarial, and are more like a case conference than a trial. The aim of the proceedings is to rehabilitate the doctor while maintaining patient safety. The GMC does not publicize its decision, but if a decision is made that affects registration the doctor's employer is informed. If the Committee decides on suspension or conditional registration, this will be reviewed before the due expiry date with a further medical examination and reports from the medical supervisor on the doctor's progress. The Health Committee has no power to strike the doctor off the register. However, if the doctor is given two consecutive one-year suspensions, the Committee can suspend registration indefinitely, subject to appeal by the doctor himself.

Part 6

Doctors' Rights

Chapter 18

Employment and other rights of doctors

It might seem strange to end a book on medical ethics and law by considering the rights of doctors. However, it seems to us that doctors have essentially two sets of rights (Table 18.1), and these are sometimes perhaps overlooked.

First, they have a right to act ethically and to be respected for acting in good faith and with integrity. They should have access to the resources to provide the best available treatment for their patients. They have a right to respect and consideration and to be free from undue interference whilst undertaking their clinical duties. They have a right to professional integrity and freedom. Second, doctors have a right to proper conditions of service and employment.

Right (and duty) to act ethically

It is perhaps self-evident that if doctors have duties toward patients, they have a right to act ethically and to have the means to be able to fulfil their obligations towards those patients.

Patients expect their doctors to 'act in good faith'. Often patients will ask 'What would you do, doctor?' or 'Do you think this treatment is right for me?' A lot of the communication between doctors and patients is non-verbal. Patients will gain much not just from what the doctor says, but from how it is said. This is particularly true in the context of palliative care, 'breaking bad news' or discussing matters when there has been a medical mishap.

Does the doctor show concern, are they worried by the patient's condition, are they evasive? Do they answer questions simply and clearly? Can the doctor be trusted? These are important patient-centred questions that doctors must face.

The rights of doctors with conscientious objections must be respected. Doctors must not be forced to act against their honestly held beliefs. Avenues of practice should not be barred because of conscientiously held views (Table 18.2).

In the Hippocratic tradition, doctors are expected to act ethically, and this was the measure of the respect owed to the physician.

'If I fulfil this oath and do not violate it, may it be granted to me to enjoy life and [my] art, being honoured with fame among all men for all time to come; if I transgress it and swear falsely, may the opposite of all this be my lot.'
Hippocratic *Oath* (translation from the Greek by Ludwig Edelstein, 1943)

It is the job of organizations like the BMA and the GMC (the statutory body) to ensure that government is sufficiently well advised about medical ethical issues that no attempt is made to undermine the profession by any law that clashes with fundamental medical ethics or that places doctors in a professionally embarrassing position or undermines the doctor–patient relationship of trust.

It is, primarily, the underlying purpose of medical ethics to foster that trust by enabling the

Table 18.1 Rights of a doctor

Right (and duty) to act ethically
- To exercise proper clinical judgement
- To act as patient advocate for the benefit of the individual
- To act 'in good faith'
- To exercise a right of conscientious objection in contentious cases such as abortion
- To respect and consideration in dealing with their patients
- To academic freedom in conducting ethical research
- To professional autonomy and self-regulation to a reasonable extent and so far as the law allows

Employment rights
- Employment rights under the law
- Access to complaints procedures
- Protection when 'whistle blowing'
- Right to a fair trial regarding complaints against the doctor
- To freedom from interference, harassment and unmeritorious complaints
- Freedom from bullying and harassment in the workplace

Table 18.2 BMA advice on conscientious objection to abortion

The BMA Ethics Committee amended its guidance on abortion following a resolution of the Annual Representative Meeting in 1999 that stated that it abhorred the harassment of doctors 'who conscientiously object to participation in termination of pregnancy'.

In *The Law and Ethics of Abortion: BMA Views*, the Committee has added the following:

'Some doctors have complained of being harassed and discriminated against because of their conscientious objection to termination of pregnancy. The association abhors such behaviour and any BMA members who feel they are being pressured to participate in terminations of pregnancy contrary to their conscience, or are being harassed in this way, should contact their regional office for advice and support.'

BMJ 1999; 319:925

public to feel that they can have confidence in the profession because it will always maintain the highest standards, medically, ethically and in every way.

Employment rights and the law

The doctor has two contracts:
- A professional contract with the individual patient.
- A contractual arrangement either with an employer, or, in the case of private practice, with the patient.

Hospital doctors will have a contract to provide services within the NHS. Their rights are protected under employment law.

The professional contract with the patient is governed by the rules laid down by the GMC. However, all NHS contracts require the doctor to be registered with the GMC, and NHS organizations expect doctors to abide by GMC professional guidelines.

The European Working Time Directive

The contracts for consultants, medical academics and GPs have recently been re-negotiated. It is not possible to go into any detail about these contracts here. However, the working time directive (EWTD) applies to doctors, including junior doctors in training (Table 18.3). Compliance with the European Working Time Directive is part of our treaty obligations as members of the European Union.

The meaning of 'work time' according to the Directive is:

'any period during which the worker is working, at the employer's disposal and carrying out his activity or duties, in accordance with national laws and/or practice'.

The European Court of Justice was asked to decide on whether time on call could be regarded as working time, and decided that only time spent actually working or time on the premises would be working time. Being non-resident on call would not constitute working.

Table 18.3 What is the European Working Time Directive (EWTD)?

The EWTD is part of European Law. It came into domestic UK law in 1988 under Article 138 of the European Treaty in order to protect the health and safety of employees.

Doctors in training were initially excluded from the Directive. However a transition timetable (Table 18.4) has been introduced for junior doctors after a compromise between the position of the European Parliament, which had wanted the EWTD to apply to juniors within 4 years, and the Council of Ministers, which had wanted implementation within 13 years.

Table 18.4 Expected timetable for implementation of the European Working Time Directive

August 2004	Interim 58-hour maximum working week. Rest and break requirements apply from this date.
August 2007	Maximum 56-hour working week
August 2009	Deadline for 48-hour maximum. This may exceptionally be extended for another 3 years, with an interim week of 52 hours, with the 48-hour week coming in 2012.

Table 18.5 Rest and break periods under the EWTD

- A maximum average working week of 48 hours including overtime.
- A minimum daily consecutive rest period of 11 hours.
- A minimum rest break of 20 minutes when the working day exceeds 6 hours.
- A minimum rest period of 24 hours in each seven-day period.
- A minimum of 4 weeks paid annual leave.
- A maximum of 8 hours work in any 24 hours for night workers in stressful jobs.

'Time spent on call by doctors . . . must be regarded in its entirety as working time . . . if they are required to be present at the health centre. If they must merely be contactable at all times when on call, only time linked to the actual provision of . . . services must be regarded as working time.'

Sindicato de Medicos de Asistencia Publica (SIMAP) — v — Conselleria de Sanidad y Consumo de la Generalidad Valenciana, Case C- 303/98 (2000).

The definition of work in the SIMAP case has recently been confirmed in the *Jaeger* case in September 2003. Time spent resident on call for clinical purposes is regarded as 'working time' in its entirety. Put simply, doctors resident on call but asleep are to be counted as working, which is good news for junior doctors. When a doctor is not resident on call, however, only time actually spent working is regarded as working time.

Members of staff may choose to opt out of the EWTD provided that they sign a waiver. The employee may opt in again subject to an agreed period of notice. There is no compulsion to opt out. However, doctors cannot opt out of the requirements for rest periods. Nevertheless, because of the nature of clinical work, where rest cannot be taken, compensatory rest periods should be taken within a reasonable period of time and within the normal working week.

Doctors in training will be subject to the provisions of the EWTD from August 2004, when the transitional working-time hours limits will apply (Table 18.4).

The hours of work under the EWTD for a maximum 48-hour week are shown in Table 18.5.

Protection from the consequences of 'whistle-blowing'

An employee may take his employer to a tribunal for unfair dismissal or redundancy after a disclosure ('whistle-blowing'):
- in relation to a criminal offence
- in relation to a breach of a legal obligation, e.g. a duty of care
- where the health and safety of an employee is likely to be endangered, for example by bullying
- where there has been a miscarriage of justice
- where there has been environmental damage.

An employee may also disclose information where it is otherwise likely to be concealed, provided that the worker:

Table 18.6 A definition of bullying

A useful definition of bullying is:
'Persistent, offensive, abusive, intimidating, malicious or insulting behaviour, abuse of power or unfair penal sanctions, which makes the recipient feel upset, threatened, humiliated or vulnerable, which undermines their self-confidence and which may cause them to suffer stress.'

Lyons R, Tivey H, Ball C. *Bullying at work: how to tackle it. A guide for MSF representatives and members.* London: MSF, 1995

Table 18.7 Characteristics of bullying

Categories of bullying behaviour:
1 **Threat to professional status**
   - belittling opinion, public humiliation, accusations of poor effort
2 **Threat to personal standing**
   - insults, verbal abuse, teasing
3 **Isolation**
   - denying teaching opportunities, withholding information
4 **Overwork**
   - undue pressure of work, impossible deadlines, unnecessary interruptions
5 **Destabilization**
   - failing to give credit, meaningless tasks, removing responsibility, shifting 'goal posts'.

Rayner C, Hoel H. 'A summary review of literature relating to workplace bullying'. *J Comm Appl Soc Psychol.* 1997; 7: 181–91.

- reasonably believes it to be true;
- does not make the revelation for personal gain;
- does not commit any offence by making the disclosure, e.g. does not breach the Official Secrets Act.

Freedom from bullying and harassment

Bullying and harassment is not as uncommon as it should be within the NHS. Many junior doctors experience some form of bullying. In one study of SHOs and Registrars, it was found that up to 37% of junior doctors reported bullying within the previous year. Black and Asian doctors were more likely to be bullied than white doctors, and women were more frequently bullied than men (Lyn Quine, 2002).

Despite being self-reported episodes from a survey with only a 59% response rate, the findings are disturbing, and would be consistent with high rates of bullying in the workplace generally.

Bullying is defined in terms of the effects on the recipient, not of the intention of the bully. It must have a negative effect on the victim. Bullying behaviour must be persistent. The characteristics of bullying and the way it may affect the victim are outlined in Table 18.7.

UK and EC Law in relation to bullying and harassment

There is no specific law in relation to bullying, so that cases are brought in relation to a number of different laws. Harassment may involve a number of issues, including breach of contract, personal injury, including psychiatric injury, negligence, malicious falsehood, manslaughter (where bullying has led to suicide), breach of natural justice, when employers act as 'judge and jury', and even contempt of court, when employees acting as witnesses are intimidated to withdraw or retract statements under threat of loosing their jobs.

Unfair conduct against an employee may give rise to a claim for constructive dismissal in the Employment Tribunal, even though no actual dismissal has occurred, and discrimination claims, e.g. on the basis of race or sex, may be brought in the Employment Tribunal or the County Court.

Harassment may be criminal, and may be prosecuted under the Protection from Harassment Act 1997 (the so-called 'anti-stalking' Act) or may give rise to a civil claim for an injunction to prevent harassment.

Harassment is defined in s.2 of the 1997 Act as being where

'a reasonable person in possession of the same information would think the course of conduct amounted to harassment of the other';

and s.1 makes it an offence to pursue a course of

conduct amounting to harassment that the defendant

'knows or ought to know amounts to harassment of the other'.

Information and references

The House of Lords in *Spring v. Corinium and* *Guardian Assurance* (1994) held that employers are under a duty to take reasonable care in the preparation of a reference, and would be liable if it proved to be inaccurate and the employee were to suffer damage as a consequence.

Doctors also have a right under the Data Protection Act 1998 to information held about them.

Philosophers who have influenced medical ethics

AQUINAS, Thomas (1224–74). He is generally regarded as one of the greatest medieval theologians. He was schooled at the monastery of Monte Cassino and studied liberal arts at the University of Naples, where he was introduced to the works of Aristotle through the writings of the Islamic philosopher Averroes. He became a pupil of Albertus Magnus (Albert the Great) and studied at the University of Paris from 1254 to 1259. Aquinas attempted to produce a synthesis of Christian thought and Aristotelianism. His written output was enormous, and includes two massive treatises on philosophy and theology—the *Summa contra Gentiles* and the *Summa Theologica*. He wrote a number of commentaries on the works of Aristotle, including commentaries on the *Analytics*, *De Anima*, *De Caelo*, the *Ethics*, *De Interpretatione*, the *Metaphysics and* the *Politics*. He extended the Aristotelian concepts of the nature of happiness, virtue, human action, free will, and intention and applied them to the concepts of divine law and grace.

ARISTOTLE (384–322 BC). He was born at Stagirus in Chalcidice and his father was court physician to the King of Macedonia. He entered Plato's Academy at the age of 17 and remained there for 20 years, as student and teacher, until Plato's death. He then left Athens and became tutor to the young Alexander the Great. He later returned to Athens and founded the Lyceum, where he taught for the next 12 years. Following the death of Alexander he was forced to flee Athens and took refuge in Euboea, where he died shortly afterwards. In addition to his philosophical and metaphysical writings, he wrote major works on logic (*Logical Works*, *The Categories*, *Prior and Posterior Analytics*, *Topics and Sophistical Fallacies*), physical sciences (the *Physics*, *On Motion*, *On Astronomy*, *On Magnets*, *Meteorology*), biological sciences (*Researches*, *Dissections* (seven books), *On Plants, the History of Animals*—ten books on comparative anatomy and physiology, although one is probably post-Aristotelian), psychology (*De Anima*), politics (*Lectures on Political Theory*—eight books, *Politics*, the *Constitution of Athens*), ethics (*Magna Moralia*, *Nicomachean Ethics* and *Eudemian Ethics*) as wells as works on aesthetics, history, literature and the arts (*Rhetoric*, *Poetics*). In addition to these major works he also wrote on perception, memory, sleeping and waking, dreams, long life and short life, life and death and divination in sleep. Aristotle undertook original research and first-hand study, making his own observations and carrying out his own dissections. For example, in the *Researches* he describes the early development of embryonic chicks from eggs.

AVERROES (Ibn Rushd) (1126–98). Islamic philosopher, doctor and judge who spent most of his life in Seville and Cordova, Spain. He wrote numerous philosophical treatises, including commentaries on Aristotle as well as on jurisprudence and medicine. As a rationalist, he held that the Qur'an was allegorical, and he was critical of mysticism and disagreed with Avicenna on the nature of the Deity. The influence of Averroes on Islamic thought was less than that on medieval Europe, especially after many of his commentaries were translated from Arabic into Latin in the thirteenth century.

AVICENNA (Ibn Sina) (980–1037). Islamic philosopher who also made substantial contributions to medicine, science and mathematics. He wrote the first study of Aristotle in Persian, and wrote over 200 works. He held that philosophy and religion are harmonious and that Islam is the highest mode of human life. Only in God do essence and existence coincide. His main works were *The Book of Healing (of the Soul)*, *The Book of Salvation* and *The Canon of Medicine*. His medical works remained standard sources of knowledge for centuries.

AYER, Alfred J. (1910–1989). Wykeham Professor of Logic at Oxford (1959), knighted in 1970. His *Language, Truth and Logic* (1936) outlined the theory of logical positivism of the Vienna Circle. Logical positivism deals with problems of reality, perception, induction, knowledge and meaning. According to Ayer, philosophy is a means of analysis. Since metaphysical truths can neither be confirmed nor refuted by philosophical investigation, they are meaningless. Professor Ayer espoused emotivism—the theory that moral statements are neither true nor false but rather expressions of emotional reactions in much the same way as crying at bad news or laughing at jokes. Fundamental ethical concepts are essentially unanalysable, as there is no criterion of validity. Moral precepts are mere pseudo-concepts. Ayer's conclusions about ethics applied equally to aesthetics, and words like 'beautiful' and 'hideous' are employed in the same way that ethical words are.

BENTHAM, Jeremy (1748–1832). He was the founder of Utilitarianism. His embalmed body can still be viewed at University College, London. Since 'Nature has placed mankind under the governance of two sovereign masters, pain and pleasure' he argued that actions should be judged morally right or wrong according to whether or not they maximized pleasure and minimized pain. He established the 'greatest happiness principle', whereby the measure of ethics was that which provided the greatest happiness to the greatest number. Utilitarianism removes duties, rules and values, and bases morality on the consequences of actions, where 'each is to count for one and none for more than one'. Bentham also wrote extensively on matters relating to social, educational and legal reform.

DARWIN, Charles (1809–1882). His theory of evolution, set out in the *Origin of Species* (1859) and *The Descent of Man* (1871), argued that all living things evolved from simpler forms through a process of natural selection. The evolution of man was no exception. Evolutionary theory was at odds with a literal interpretation of the biblical account of creation, and was to have a profound influence on later secular ethical theories. According to Darwinian theory, man does not exist for any specific purpose but has evolved through natural selection and random mutation over millions of years. For some neo-Darwinians, like Professor Richard Dawkins, there is no place for theories of morality, which are based upon the Aristotelian view that moral rules can be deduced from knowledge of the purpose or teleology of human nature.

DESCARTES, René (1596–1650). A French philosopher and mathematician, his ambition was to reconstruct philosophy anew rather than to contribute to the existing body of knowledge. Mathematical certainty was to be the paradigm for this new knowledge. He wrote: 'Those who are seeing this strict way of truth should not trouble themselves about any object concerning which they cannot have a certainty equal to arithmetical or geometrical demonstration.' He is famous for his conclusion: 'I think, therefore I am.'

HIPPOCRATES (460–377 BC). He was a Physician in ancient Greece and is called the 'Father of Medicine'. He based his practice on observations and the belief that all illness had a physical and rational explanation, rejecting the notion that disease arose form the disfavour of the Gods or possession by evil spirits. At the same time the followers of Asclepius, the God of Healing (who had been a physician around 1200 BC before he began to be regarded as a god) believed that diseases had supernatural causes and cures. Hippocrates accurately described a number of diseases, including pneumonia and epilepsy. Therapeutics were limited in his time, and Hippocrates believed in the healing properties of nature, rest, diet, fresh air and cleanliness. He travelled throughout Greece and founded a medical school on the island of Cos. The code of ethics ascribed to Hippocrates has remained the best-known code of practice for doctors in the intervening 25 centuries. The 'Hippocratic corpus' or collection of writings comprises over sixty treatises, mostly written between about 430 and 330 BC. They give a fascinating insight into ancient Greek medicine, and some of the works have been quoted in the text—*Epidemics*, *Aphorisms*, *Precepts* and *Decorum*.

HOBBES, Thomas (1588–1679). While perhaps best known for his political theories, Hobbes has also been regarded as the founding father of metaphysical materialism. Talk of incorporeal spiritual entities such as God and the human soul was, he believed, incoherent. Hence it was absurd, 'when a man is dead and buried', for anyone to say that 'his soul (that is his life) can walk separated from his body, and is seen by night amongst the graves' (*Leviathan*, Chapter 46). For Hobbes, the whole Universe is mechanical, and the human body can be regarded simply as a machine.

HUME, David (1711–76). He was a Scottish philosopher and historian, who never held an academic post, having applied unsuccessfully for the chairs at Edinburgh and Glasgow. While his *History of England* constituted the bulk of his writings, his political essays, together with those of Locke and Montesquieu, influenced the founding fathers of the US Constitution. He was a friend of Adam Smith, the influential economist. He wrote four major philosophical works: *A Treatise of Human Nature, An Inquiry concerning Human Understanding, An Inquiry concerning the Principles of Morals* and *The Dialogues concerning*

Natural Religion. He was too cautious to publish the last two in his lifetime, and they were published posthumously by his nephew. In the *Inquiry* he adopts an aggressive agnosticism about religion, and was scathing about the proofs of the existence of God. In the *Treatise* he argued that we cannot found a knowledge of the external world on our sensory experience. He talked of 'perceptions of the mind', which he divided into 'impressions' (primary) and 'ideas' (derivative). Nevertheless, we are aware mainly of the 'appearances' in our minds rather than objects in the external world. He accepted the Newtonian view that there are no really coloured objects, but rather physical objects and light rays that have 'a certain power and disposition to stir up a sensation that is colour'. Hume argued that the same applies to virtue and vice, beauty and ugliness. It was not possible to prove moral beliefs. Hume's view of moral philosophy is sometimes called 'Subjectivism'.

KANT, Immanuel (1724–1804). Born in Königsberg, Kant never left the town, and in 1770 became Professor of Logic and Metaphysics in the University. He once famously claimed that reading Hume had woken him from his 'dogmatic slumber'. His most important works were three *Critiques*—the *Critique of Pure Reason* (1781), *Critique of Practical Reason* (1788) and *Critique of Judgement* (1790). Kant argued that there are two sources of human knowledge: sensibility and understanding. He wrote: 'throughout the former, objects are given to us; throughout the latter, they are thought'. In Kant's view, understanding is the means whereby our sense data become ordered and give us an experience of an objective world. He further wrote: 'the order and regularity of objects, which we title nature, we ourselves introduce. The understanding is itself the lawgiver of nature.' For Kant, the fact of self-awareness assumes knowledge of an objective outer world; thus 'the mere consciousness of my own existence proves the existence of objects in space outside me'. Kant's most famous contribution to moral philosophy is his categorical imperative, which attempts to universalize moral principles. 'Act only on that maxim which you can at the same time will to become universal law', wrote Kant. The 'categorical' imperative is in contrast with a 'hypothetical' imperative that is contingent upon a particular aim, e.g. 'go to bed early if you want to wake refreshed in the morning'. However, for Kant, morality does not depend upon particular wishes or inclinations, since they are not, he claimed, subject to the will. Nor can actions be judged by consequences, since the results may not turn out as anticipated or desired. Rather, to act morally is to act for the sake of duty. In his third *Critique*, Kant regards the purposiveness in Nature as an unprovable but 'special *a priori* concept'. This 'teleological judgement' is an assumption that, says Kant, enables scientists to integrate particular laws into more general laws of science.

LOCKE, John (1632–1704). A highly influential philosopher whose writings formed the basis of classic empiricism and liberal democracy. He studied chemistry and medicine at Oxford and became a don at Christ Church in 1656. He was an acquaintance of Robert Boyle, with whom he shared his views on empiricism and experimental methodology, and was a friend of Isaac Newton. In 1667 he left Oxford to become personal physician to Lord Ashley, later first Earl of Shaftesbury. He later collaborated in the research of the great physician, Thomas Sydenham. His *Essay Concerning Human Understanding* (1690) is a critical assessment of the nature, origins and limits of human reason in the empirical idiom. It took into account the contemporary advances in science, and formed the base for the empiricism of Berkeley and Hume. The task of the philosopher, for Locke, was to clear 'some of the rubbish that lies in the way of knowledge'. The acquisition of knowledge he left to scientists such as Boyle and Newton. He held that there are no innate ideas, and all knowledge is derived from experience. Ideas can either be simple ideas, which have no other ideas contained within them, such as the notion of yellow or hot, or complex ideas, which are constructed out of simple ideas. Complex ideas do not necessarily correspond to reality, e.g. the idea of a unicorn. Locke distin-

guished between the primary and secondary qualities of physical things. Primary qualities are found in all bodies, such as solidity and extension in space. Secondary qualities are powers in the object that produce ideas in us such as colour, taste and smell. Locke recognized the importance of knowledge obtained through intuition. In agreement with Descartes, he taught that we can have intuitive knowledge of our own existence. We also know things through deduction or demonstration. He held it is possible to demonstrate the existence of God. He differed from Descartes in denying that we can have certain knowledge of the world, and held that scientific knowledge was at best only highly probable, rather than certain. His *Two Treatises of Government* (1690) were attempts to justify constitutional rule and the liberty of the individual. In the state of nature all men are free and equal, he wrote. However, said Locke, freedom does not mean licence, and there is a law of nature, ordained by God, by which behaviour should be regulated. We have natural rights such as the right to life and liberty, so long as our actions do not infringe the rights of others. A man has a right to private property only in so far as he has use of it. However, in order to safeguard natural rights, men must join together in a social contract under a government that enforces laws to protect their rights and adjudicate disputes. Majority rule should prevail in matters that do not infringe natural rights. His commitment to natural rights, the rule of law, the role of the state as guarantor of natural rights and majority rule were to be highly influential not only in the development of the British constitution after the Revolution of 1688 but later, after his death, in the formation of the American Constitution.

MACINTYRE, Alasdair (1929–••). An American philosopher teaching at the University of Notre Dame. It is not easy to classify Alasdair MacIntyre's philosophy. He was a Marxist, who was later strongly influenced by Wittgenstein, and later again became Christian, and draws inspiration from Aristotle and Aquinas. He is a social critic and, in particular, a critic of modern libertarianism. Central to his view is the notion that social dislocation and the moral impoverishment brought about by the libertarian individualism of the Enlightenment period has left us with a collection of moral ideas that can no longer provide us with moral guidance. According to MacIntyre, arguments about just war, abortion, capital punishment, or equality simply result in shrill and sterile debate in a postmodern intellectual climate. The remedy is a return to the Aristotelian tradition of virtue ethics. His books include *A Short History of Ethics* (1965), *After Virtue* (1981), and *Whose Justice? Which Rationality?* (1988).

PLATO (427–347 BC). It is Plato who has perhaps the greatest claim to the title of the founding father of philosophy. He was Socrates' pupil for about 10 years up to the time of Socrates' death. Plato held that it was possible to distinguish knowledge from mere opinion, that there was an objective basis to morality and that the soul was distinct from the human body and was immortal. Despite often poetic and mystical writings he raised highly practical issues in education and politics. He believed that true knowledge would enable people to live well.

SIDGWICK, Henry (1838–1900). He was a philosopher who taught at Cambridge, becoming Professor of Moral Philosophy from 1883 to1900. His most influential book was *The Method of Ethics* (1874), in which he proposed that the promotion of the general happiness (utilitarianism) was justified on the basis of a fundamental moral intuition and that a common-sense morality was generally justifiable. Reconciliation of individual self-interest and morality would require a belief in God that would be natural but rationally indefensible.

SINGER, Peter (1946–••). He is currently Professor of Bioethics at the University of Princeton. He was the author of *Animal Liberation* (1975) and is credited as one of the founders of the Animal Liberation Movement. Other major works include: *Practical Ethics* (1979), *The Reproduction Revolution*, *Should the Baby Live?* and *Rethinking Life and Death* (1995). *The New Yorker* once described him as 'the most influential living philosopher', while some of his critics regard him as 'the most dangerous man in the world'. Professor Singer is a philosophical utilitarian who has argued that animals have rights. He proposed that the issue is not whether a being can talk but whether it can suffer. He has jettisoned the traditional distinction between humans and non-humans, and distinguishes between persons and non-persons. He has proposed that foetuses and some very handicapped humans are not persons, and have a lesser moral status than adult gorillas and chimpanzees. Singer argues that it is only parents, not the state, who should decide the fate of disabled infants.

STUART MILL, John (1806–1836). A philosopher and social reformer, he was educated by his father, James Mill, who was a disciple of Bentham. In *Utilitarianism* (1863) he modified Bentham's ethics by regarding self-interest as an inadequate criterion of goodness, and by making qualitative distinctions between types of pleasure. *On Liberty* (1859) related the freedoms of individuals—belief, tastes and pursuits, and uniting with others—to the powers of authority and social demands. In Mill's view, restrictions on the freedom of individuals were justified only to prevent actual harm to others.

Appendix 2

Suggested further reading

Chapter 1. Nature and origins of medical ethics

'Medical Professionalism in the New Millennium: A Physician Charter: Project of the ABIM Foundation, ACP-ASMIM Foundation and European Federation of Internal Medicine', *Ann Intern Med*, 2002;136:243–6.

Aristotle, *The Nicomachean Ethics*, translated by W. D. Ross, Oxford University Press, London, 1959.

Beauchamp, Tom, and Childress, James, *Principles of Biomedical Ethics*, 5th edn, New York, Oxford University Press, 2001.

Hippocratic Writings, edited by G. E. R. Lloyd (Penguin Classics), Penguin Books, Harmondsworth, 1983. [Excerpts from the Hippocratic writings, including passages from *Epidemics*, *Aphorisms*, *Precepts* and *Decorum*.]

British Medical Association, *Medical Ethics Today*. BMJ Books, London, 2004. [The BMA's handbook on ethics and law.]

The Islamic Code of Medical Ethics, Kuwait 1981 can be found on the internet at *www.islamset.com/ethics/code/index.html*

Chapter 2. Sources of medical law

The Human Rights Act 1998 can be accessed on the web at: *www.hmso.gov.uk/acts/acts1998/19980042.htm*

Kennedy, I., and Grubb, A., *Medical Law*. Butterworth, London, 2000.

Mason, J. K., McCall Smith, R. A., and Laurie, G. T., *Law and Medical Ethics*, 6th edn, Butterworth, London, 2002.

NB: See Appendix 3 for a brief introduction to looking up the law.

Chapter 3. Consent to treatment

GMC, *Seeking patient's consent: the ethical considerations*. GMC, 178 Great Portland Street. London W1N 6JE, 1998.

The Law Society and the BMA, *Assessment of Mental Capacity. Guidance for doctors and lawyers*. BMA, London, 1995.

Chapter 4. Confidentiality

The Caldicott Report (1997). Published by the Department of Health. *http://www.doh.gov.uk/ipu/confiden/report/index.htm*

GMC, *Confidentiality: protecting and providing information*. GMC, 178 Great Portland Street. London W1N 6JE, September 2000.

Chapter 5. Clinical negligence

Kennedy, I., and Grubb, A., *Medical Law*. Butterworth, London, 2000.

Mason, J. K., McCall Smith, R. A., and Laurie, G. T., *Law and Medical Ethics*, 6th edn, Butterworth, London, 2002.

Making Amends. The Chief Medical Officer's Report can be accessed on the website at: *http://www.doh.gov.uk/makingamends/pdf*

Civil Procedure Rules. http://www.dca.gov.uk/civil/procrules_fin/menus/rules.htm

See in particular:

Part 1 — the Overriding Objective — *http://www.dca.gov.uk/civil/procrules_fin/contents/parts/part01.htm*

Part 2 — Application and Interpretation of the Rules — *http://www.dca.gov.uk/civil/procrules_fin/contents/parts/part02.htm*

Part 3 — The Court's Case Management Powers — *http://www.dca.gov.uk/civil/procrules_fin/contents/parts/part03.htm*

Part 7 — How to Start Proceedings *http://www.dca.gov.uk/civil/procrules_fin/contents/parts/part07.htm*

Part 9 — Responding to Particulars of Claim — General *http://www.dca.gov.uk/civil/procrules_fin/contents/parts/part09.htm*

Pre-action Protocols for the Resolution of Clinical Disputes *http://www.dca.gov.uk/civil/procrules_fin/contents/protocols/prot_rcd.htm*

Chapter 6. Mental health

Jones, Richard, *Mental Health Act Manual*. 8th edn, Sweet and Maxwell, London, 2002.

Chapter 8. The law in relation to abortion

GMC, *Professional conduct and discipline: fitness to practise*. GMC, 178 Great Portland Street. London W1N 6JE, February 1991.

Shapira, A., 'Wrongful life lawsuits for faulty genetic counselling: should the impaired newborn be entitled to sue?' *J Med Ethics*. 1998. Dec;24(6):369–75.

Gillon, R., 'Wrongful life claims'. *J Med Ethics*. 1998. Dec;24(6):363–364.

Dorozynski, A., 'Highest French court awards compensation for "being born" ', *BMJ*, 2001. Dec;15:323.

Chapter 9. The ethics of abortion

GMC, *Professional conduct and discipline: fitness to practise*. GMC, 178 Great Portland Street. London W1N 6JE, February 1991.

Nathanson, B. N. and Ostling, R. N., *Aborting America*, Doubleday & Co., New York, 1979.

Gissler, M., Kauppila, R., Merilainen, J., Toukomaa, H., and Elina Hemminki, E., 'Pregnancy-associated deaths in Finland 1987–1994 — definition problems and benefits of record linkage', *Acta Obstet Gyn Scand* 76(1997):651–7.

Gissler, M., Berg, C., Bouvier-Colle, M. H., and Buekens, P., 'Pregnancy-associated mortality after birth, spontaneous abortion or induced abortion in Finland, 1987–2000', *Am J Ob Gyn* 2004;190:422–7.

Reardon, D. C., Ney, P. G., Scheuren, F., Cougle, J., Coleman, P. K., and Strahan, T. W., 'Deaths associated with pregnancy outcome: a record linkage study of low income women', *South Med J* 2002 Aug;95(8):834–41.

Bousingen, D. D., 'France tightens disabled patients' rights to sue doctors', *Lancet* 2002;359(9302):233.

Reardon, D. C., Cougle, J. R., Shuping, M. W., Coleman, P. K., and Ney, P. G., 'Psychiatric admissions of low-income women following abortion and childbirth', *Canadian Medical Association Journal* 2003;168(10):1253–6.

Morgan, C. L., Evans, M., Peters, J. R., and Currie, C., 'Suicide after pregnancy', *BMJ* 1997;314:902.

Brind, J. *et al.*, 'Induced abortion as an independent risk factor for breast cancer: a comprehensive review and meta-analysis', *J Epidemiology and Community Health*, 1996;50:481–96.

Royal College of Obstetricians and Gynaecologists, *Breast Cancer and Pregnancy Guideline number 12*, January 2004.

Collaborative Group on Hormonal Factors in Breast Cancer, 'Breast Cancer and abortion: collaborative re-analysis of data from 53 epidemiological studies, including 83,000 women with breast cancer from 16 countries.', *Lancet* 2004;363:1007–16.

Chapter 10. Reproductive technology and surrogacy

Human Embryology and Fertilization Authority. Patient Information. *www.hfea.gov.uk*

Chapter 11. The law in relation to end-of-life issues

Department of Health, *Diagnosis of brain stem death including guidelines for the identification and management of potential organ and tissue donors*, March 1998. *http://doh.gov.uk/pdfs/ brainstemdeath.pdf*

Royal College of Physicians Working Group, 'The permanent vegetative state. Review by a working group convened by the Royal College of Physicians and endorsed by the Conference of Medical Royal Colleges and their faculties of the United Kingdom', *J Royal Coll Physicians*, London, 1996;30:119–21.

A consensus statement on criteria for the persistent vegetative state is being developed. See the letter of Jennett, B., Crandford, R., and Zasler, N., *BMJ* 1997;314:1621, quoting the original paper describing PVS: Jennet, B., and Plum F., 'Persistent vegetative state after brain damage; a syndrome in search of a name', *Lancet* 1972;I:734–7.

Andrews, K., Murphy, L., Munday, R., and Littlewood, C., 'Misdiagnosis of the vegetative state: retrospective study in a rehabilitation unit', *BMJ* 1996:313–16.

Chapter 12. The ethics of end-of-life issues

Decisions Relating to Cardiopulmonary Resuscitation. A joint statement from the British Medical Association, the Resuscitation Council (UK) and the Royal College of Nursing. March 2001. The purpose of these guidelines is to outline legal and ethical standards for planning patient care and decision-making in relation to cardiopulmonary resuscitation.

Resuscitation policy (HSC 2000/028). NHS Executive. London. Department of Health, September 2000.

Resuscitation policy (HDL (2000) 22). Scottish Health Department. Edinburgh: Scottish Executive, November 2000.

Chapter 13. Clinical research

Burleigh, Michael, *Death and Deliverance: Euthanasia in Germany 1900–1945*, Cambridge University Press, Cambridge, 1994.

World Medical Association Declaration of Helsinki. 'Ethical Principles for Medical Research Involving Human Subjects', 52nd WMA General Assembly, Edinburgh, October 2000. Note on clarification of paragraph 29 added by the WMA General Assembly, Washington, 2002.

The use of human organs and tissue: an interim report. DOH April 2003. *www.dog.gov.uk 'tissue' interimstatment.pdf*

Chapter 14. Maintaining standards and professional regulation

Learning from Bristol: the report of the public inquiry into children's heart surgery at the Bristol Royal Infirmary 1984–1995. Command Paper CM 5207 (I). HMSO 2001. *http://www.bristol-inquiry.org.uk*

Chapter 15. Presenting evidence and rules of procedure

Berlins, Marcel and Dyer, Clare, *The Law Machine*, 5th edn, Penguin Books, Harmondsworth, 2000.

Civil Procedure Rules. http://www.dca.gov.uk/civil/ procrules_fin/menus/rules.htm

See in particular:

Part 1—the Overriding Objective—*http://www.dca. gov.uk/civil/procrules_fin/contents/parts/part01.htm*

Part 2—Application and Interpretation of the Rules—*http://www.dca.gov.uk/civil/ procrules_fin/contents/puits/part02.htm*

Part 3—The Court's Case Management Powers—*http://www.dca.gov.uk/civil/procrules_fin/contents/ parts/part03.htm*

Part 35—Experts and Assessors—*http://www.dca. gov.uk/civil/procrules_fin/contents/parts/part35.htm*

Chapter 17. The General Medical Council

GMC, *Good Medical Practice*, 3rd edn, GMC, 178 Great Portland Street, London W1N 6JE, 2001. *http://www.gmc-uk.org/standards/good.htm*

GMC, *Tomorrow's Doctors. Recommendations on undergraduate medical education*, GMC, 178 Great Portland Street, London W1N 6JE, 2003. *http://www.gmc-uk.org/med_ed/tomdoc.htm*

Implementing the New Doctor: the Education Committee's informal visits to UK universities. October 1998 to April 2001. GMC. 2002. *http://www.gmc-uk.org/med_ed/itnd.htm*

Chapter 18. Employment and other rights of doctors

Doctors in training and the European Working Time Directive—the current legal position, RCP London. Available at: *http://www.rcplondon.ac.uk/college/statements/doc_ewtd_legal.asp*

Quine, L., 'Workplace bullying in NHS community trust: staff questionnaire survey', *BMJ* 1999;318(7178):228–32.

McAvoy, B. R., and Murtagh, J., 'Workplace bullying', *BMJ* 2003;326(7393):776–7.

Dooley, D., (Editorial), 'Conscientious refusal to assist with abortion', *BMJ* 1994;309:622–3.

Beecham, L., 'BMA amends guidance on abortion', *BMJ* 1999;319:925.

World Medical Association Declaration on Physician Independence and Professional Freedom. WMA. October 1986.

World Medical Association Declaration on Professional Autonomy and Self-Regulation. WMA. October 1987.

How to access legal reference materials

The best course of action is to seek assistance from a librarian in a Law Library. Other librarians will be able to give you some assistance also.

In general, to look for a case or a statute it is advisable to look first in a case or statute citator e.g. *Current Law Case Citator*. This has cases listed in alphabetical order within certain date ranges, and gives the appropriate references so that the case can be located on the shelves of a law library. Remember to look the case up under the names of all parties cited if you cannot find it at first — for instance, on appeal the order of names may be reversed.

For a statute it is also important to check that it is still in force, and that can be done by referring to a work like *Is It in Force?*

Statutes and Statutory Instruments can be located in Halsbury's *Statutes* or *Statutory Instruments*, available in almost all law libraries and in the law sections of many other libraries.

There are now a bewildering variety of on-line sources of legal information of which some are included in the following:

Free

The government court service website: *http://www.courtservice.gov.uk/*

The House of Lords judicial website: *http://www.publications.parliament.uk/pa/ld199697/ldjudgmt/ldjudgmt.htm*

The Council of Europe website: *http://www.coe.int/portalT.asp*

British and Irish Legal Information Institute: *http://www.bailii.org/*

Subscriber service

The Official Law Reports service: *http://www.lawreports.co.uk/*

The All England Law Reports: *http://www.lexis-nexis.co.uk/site/All_England_Direct.asp*

Casetrack: *http://www.casetrack.com*

Lawtel: *http://www.lawtel.com*

There are many others, and these are given merely to provide a starting-point.

Knowledge of abbreviations is obviously vital to identify where law reports can be found, and a few are therefore given below:

AC = Appeal Cases of the Official Law Reports

All ER = the All England Law Reports

ALR = Australian Law Reports

BMLR = Butterworth's Medical Law Reports

CA = Court of Appeal

ChD = Chancery Division (High Court) cases of the Official Law Reports

CLR = Commonwealth Law Reports (Australia)

Crim LR = the Criminal Law Reports

Cr App Rep = the Criminal Appeal Reports

ECHR = European Court of Human Rights

EHRR = European Human Rights Reports

Fam = Family Division (High Court) cases of the Official Law Reports

Fam Law = reports in the *Family Law* journal

FCR = the Family Court Reporter

FLR = the Family Law Reports

HC (Aus) = High Court of Australia

HL = House of Lords

HRLR = Human Rights Law Reports

IH = Inner House (of the Scottish Court of Session)

JP = reports in the *Justice of the Peace* magazine

LS Gaz = the *Law Society Gazette* reports

Med LR — the Medical Law Reports

NLJR = *New Law Journal* Reports

OH = Outer House (of the Scottish Court of Session)

PIQR = Personal Injury Quarterly Reports

QB or KB = Queen's Bench or King's Bench Division (High Court) cases of the Official Law Reports

SC = Scottish Cases

Sol Jo = reports in the *Solicitors' Journal*

The Times = the law reports in *The Times* newspaper.

WLR = the *Weekly Law Reports*

Only a small selection of cases are ever reported, and they include most of the important ones. However, some are not reported, and may be very difficult to trace. Moreover, reported cases often do not appear in printed form for many months after the case has concluded.

A standardized form of case notation (neutral case citation) has therefore been adopted by the courts for referring to all cases, including those that are not reported, so that reference can be easily made to them. In England and Wales they include:

EWHC = England and Wales (High Court)

EWCA = England and Wales (Court of Appeal)

EWHL = England and Wales (House of Lords)

The date and case number is then included thus, for example:

B v an NHS Hospital Trust [2002] EWHC 429.

Appendix 4

Cases

Airedale NHS Trust v Bland [1993] AC 789; [1993] 2
WLR 316; [1993] 1 All ER 821; [1994] [1993] 1
FLR 1026; 1 FCR 485; [1993] Fam Law 473;
[1993] Crim LR 877; [1993] 4 Med LR 39; 12
BMLR 64; (1993) NLJR 199, HL.

AK, Re: [2001] 1 FLR 129; [2001] 2 FCR 35; 58
BMLR 151; [2000] Fam Law 885.

Anns v London Borough of Merton [1978] AC 728;
[1977] 2 WLR 1024; [1977] 2 All ER 492; (1987)
84 LS Gaz 319; (1987) NLJR 794, HL.

Attorney-General v Guardian Newspapers Ltd (No 2)
[1990] 1 AC 90; [1988] 3 WLR 776; [1988] 3 All
ER 545; (1988) NLJR 296, HL.

Attorney General's Reference (No 3 of 1994) [1998]
AC 245; [1997] 3 WLR 421; [1997] 3 All ER 936;
[1998] 1 Cr App Rep 91; [1997] Crim LR 829;
(1997) 36 LS Gaz R 44; (1997) NLJR 1185, HL.

B (Consent to Treatment: Capacity) Re:, sub nom *B v
NHS Hospital Trust; B (Adult: Refusal of Treatment), Re:* [2002] 2 All ER 449; [2002] 1 FLR
1090; [2002] 2 FCR 1; [2002] Lloyd's Rep Med
265; 65 BMLR 149; [2002] Fam Law 423; (2002)
17 LS Gaz 37, (2002) NLJR 470.

B v Croydon Health Authority [1995] Fam 133;
[1995] 2 WLR 294; [1995] 1 All ER 683; [1995] 1
FLR 470; [1995] 1 FCR 662; [1995] Fam Law 244;
22 BMLR 13; (1994) NLJR 1696.

Barnett v Chelsea and Kensington Hospital [1969] 1
QB 428; [1968] 2 WLR 422; [1968] 1 All ER 1068.

Barrett v Ministry of Defence [1995] 1 WLR 1217;
[1995] 3 All ER 87, CA.

Bolam v Friern Hospital Management Committee
[1957] 1 WLR 582; [1957] 2 All ER 118; 1 BMLR
1; 101 Sol Jo 357.

Bolitho v Hackney HA [1998] AC 232; [1997] 3 WLR
1151; [1997] 4 All ER 771; 39 BMLR 1; (1997) 47
LS Gaz R 30, 141 Sol Jo LB 238, HL.

*C (A Minor) (Wardship: Medical Treatment) (No 2),
Re:* [1990] Fam 39; [1989] 3 WLR 252; [1989] 2
All ER 791; [1990] 1 FLR 263; [1990] FCR 229;
[1990] Fam Law 133; (1989) NLJR 613, CA.

C (Adult: Refusal of Medical Treatment), Re: [1994] 1
WLR 290; [1994] 1 All ER 819; [1994] 1 FLR 31;
[1994] 2 FCR 151; [1994] Fam Law 131; 15
BMLR 77; (1993) NLJR 1642.

C v S [1988] QB 135; [1987] 2 WLR 1108; [1987] 1
All ER 1230; [1987] 2 FLR 505; [1987] Fam Law
269; (1987) 84 LS Gaz R 1410; 131 Sol Jo 624,
CA.

Camden LBC v R (A Minor) (Blood Transfusion) sub
nom *R (A Minor)(Medical Treatment), Re:* [1993] 2
FLR 757; [1993] 2 FCR 544; [1993] Fam Law 577;
(1994) LS Gaz 341; 137 Sol Jo 151.

Caparo Industries Plc v Dickman [1990] 2 AC 605;
[1990] 2 WLR 358; [1990] 1 All ER 568; [1990]
BCC 164; [1990] BCLC 273; (1990) 12 LS Gaz
42; (1990) NLJR 248, HL.

Cassidy v Ministry of Health [1951] 2 KB 343; [1951]
1 All ER 574; 95 Sol Jo 253; [1951] 1 TLR 539, CA.

Chester v. Afshar [2002] 3 WLR 1195; [2002] 3 All
ER 552; [2002] Lloyd's Rep Med 305; 67 BMLR
66; (2002) 29 LS Gaz 33; 146 Sol Jo 167, CA.

Chatterton v Gerson [1981] QB 432; [1980] 3 WLR
1003; [1981] 1 All ER 257; 1 BMLR 80; 124 Sol Jo
885.

Defreitas v O'Brien, sub nom *Defreitas v Connelly*
[1995] 6 Med LR 108; 25 BMLR 51; (1995) PIQR
P281.

Donoghue (or McAlister) v Stevenson [1932] AC 562;
[1932] All ER Rep 1; 76 Sol Jo 396, HL.

F, Re: (Mental Patient: Sterilisation) [1990] 2 AC 1;
[1989] 2 WLR 1025; [1989] 2 FLR 376; [1989]
Fam Law 390; (1989) NLJR 789; 133 Sol Jo 785;
sub nom *F v West Berkshire HA (Mental Health
Act Commission intervening)* [1989] 2 All ER 545;
4 BMLR 1, HL.

F (In Utero), Re: [1988] Fam 122; [1988] 2 WLR
1288; [1988] 2 All ER 193; [1988] 2 FLR 307;
[1988] FCR 529; [1988] Fam Law 337; (1988)
NLJR 37; 133 Sol Jo 1088, CA.

Fox v Riverside NHS Trust sub nom *Riverside Mental
Health NHS Trust v Fox* [1994] 1 FLR 614; [1994]
2 FCR 577; [1995] 6 Med LR 181; [1994] Fam
Law 321, CA.

Freeman v Home Office (No. 2) [1984] QB 524;
[1984] 2 WLR 802; [1984] 1 All ER 1036; (1984)
81 LS Gaz 1045; 128 Sol Jo 298, CA.

Gillick v West Norfolk and Wisbech AHA [1986] AC
112; [1985] 3 WLR 830; [1985] 3 All ER 402;
[1986] 1 FLR 224; [1986] Crim LR 113; 2 BMLR
11; (1985) 82 LS Gaz R 3531; (1985) NLJR 1055;
129 Sol Jo 738, HL.

Gregory v Pembrokeshire HA [1989] 1 Med LR 81.

Hatcher v. Black, The Times, 2 July 1954.

Hedley Byrne & Co. Ltd v Heller & Partners Ltd [1964]
AC 465; [1963] 3 WLR 101; [1963] 2 All ER 575;
[1963] Lloyd's Rep 485; 107 Sol Jo 454, HL.

Hill v Chief Constable of West Yorkshire [1989] AC
53; [1988] 2 WLR 1049; [1988] 2 All ER 238;
(1988) 20 LS Gaz 34; (1988) NLJR 126; 132 Sol
Jo 700, HL.

Home Office v Dorset Yacht Co Ltd [1970] AC 1004;
[1970] 2 WLR 1140; [1970] 2 All ER 294; [1970]
1 Lloyd's Rep 453; 114 Sol Jo 375, HL.

Hunter v Hanley [1995] SC 200; 1955 SLT 213.

Ireland v United Kingdom (A/25) (1979–80) 2 EHRR
25, ECHR.

J (A Minor) (Consent to Medical Treatment), Re: sub
nom *Re W (A Minor)(Medical Treatment: Court's*

Jurisdiction) [1993] Fam 64; [1992] 3 WLR 758;
[1998] 4 All ER 627; [1992] 3 Med LR 317;
(19920 NLJR 1124, CA.

Johnstone v. Bloomsbury HA [1992] QB 333; [1991]
2 WLR 1362; [1991] 2 All ER 293; [1991] 2 Med
LR; (1991) NLJR 271, CA.

Jones v. Manchester Corporation and others [1952] 2
QB 852; [1952] 2 All ER 125, 116 JP 412; [1952]
1 TLR 1589, CA.

K (Enduring Powers of Attorney), Re: F, Re: [1988]
ChD 310; [1988] 2 WLR 781; [1988] 1 All ER
358; [1988] 2 FLR 15; [1988] Fam Law 203;
(1987) NLJR 1039; 131 Sol Jo 1488.

Kent v Griffiths (No.3) [2001] QB 36; [2000] 2 WLR
1158; [2000] 2 All ER 474; [2000] Lloyd's Rep
Med 109; (2000) 7 LS Gaz 41; (2000) NLJR 195;
144 Sol Jo 106, CA.

Law Hospital NHS Trust v Lord Advocate 1996 SC
301; 1996 SLT 848 & 869; [1996] 2 FLR 407;
[1996] Fam Law 670; 39 BMLR 166, IH.

Leeds Teaching Hospitals NHS Trust v A & B & HFEA
[2003] EWHC 259.

MB (Medical Treatment), Re: [1997] 2 FLR 426;
[1997] 2 FCR 541; [1997] Fam Law 542; [1997]
8 Med LR 217; 38 BMLR 175; [1997] NLJR 600,
CA.

McCann v UK (1995) 21 EHRR 97, ECHR.

McKay v Essex AHA [1982] QB 116; [1982] 2 WLR
890; [1982] 2 All ER 771; 126 Sol Jo 261, CA.

McLelland v Greater Glasgow Health Board 2001 SLT
446; The Times, 14 Oct 1998, OH.

Margereson v Roberts [1996] PIQR P538; (1996) 22
LS Gaz 27, CA.

Maynard v West Midlands RHA [1984] 1 WLR 634;
[1985] 1 All ER 635; (1983) NLJ 641; (1984) LS
Gaz R 1926; 128 Sol Jo 317, HL.

NHS Trust A v M; NHS Trust B v H [2001] Fam 348;
[2001] 2 WLR 942; [2001] 1 All ER 801; [2001] 2
FLR 367; [2001] 1 FCR 406; [2001] HRLR 12;
[2001] Lloyd's Rep Med 28; 58 BMLR 87; [2001]
Fam Law 501

Ogwo v Taylor [1988] AC 431; [1987] 3 WLR 1145;
[1987] 3 All ER 961; (1987) NLJR 110; (1988) 4
LS Gaz 35; 131 Sol Jo 1628, HL.

Osman v UK [1999] 1 FLR 193; (2000) 29 EHRR 245;
[1999] Crim LR 82; [1999] Fam Law 86, ECHR.

Owens v Liverpool Corporation [1938] 4 All ER 727.

Paton v BPAS [1979] QB 276; [1978] 2 All ER 987; [1978] 3 WLR 687; 142 JP 497; 12 Sol Jo 744.

Penny v East Kent HA [2000] Lloyd's Rep Med 41; 55 BMLR 63; (1999) 47 LS Gaz 32; 143 Sol Jo 269.

Pigney v Pointers Transport Services Ltd [1957] 1 WLR 1121; [1957] 2 All ER 807; 101 Sol Jo 851.

Practice Note (persistent vegetative state: withdrawal of treatment) [1996] 4 All ER 766; 34 BMLR 20; sub nom *Practice Note (Official Solicitor: vegetative state)* [1996] 3 FCR 606; [1996] 2 FLR 375; [1996] Fam Law 579; (1996) NLJR 1585.

Pretty v United Kingdom (2346/02) sub nom *R (Pretty) v DPP* [2002] 2 FLR 45; [2002] 2 FCR 97; (2002) 35 EHRR 1; 66 BMLR 147; [2002] Fam Law 588; (2002) NLJR 707, ECHR.

Quintavalle v HFEA sub nom *R (Quintavalle) v HFEA* [2003] EWCA Civ 667.

R (A Child), in re [2003] EWCA Civ 182.

R (Adult: Medical Treatment), Re: [1996] 2 FLR 99; [1996] 3 FCR 473; 31 BMLR 127; [1996] Fam Law 535.

R (A Minor) (Wardship: Consent to Treatment), Re: [1992] Fam 11; [1991] 3 WLR 592; [1992] 1 FLR 190; [1992] 2 FCR 229; [1992] 3 Med LR 342; [1992] Fam Law 67, CA.

R (A Minor) (Wardship: Medical Treatment), Re: [1991] 4 All ER 177.

R v Adomako [1995] 1 AC 171; [1994] 3 WLR 288; [1994] 3 All ER 79; (1994) 99 Cr App Rep 362; 19 BMLR 56; [1994] 5 Med LR 277; [1994] Crim LR 757; (1994) NLJR 936, HL.

R v Bateman [1925] All ER 45.

R v Bourne [1939] 1 KB 687; [1938] 3 All ER 615.

R v Bournewood Community and Mental Health NHS Trust, ex.p. L sub nom L, *Re:* [1999] 1 AC 458; [1998] 3 WLR 107; [1998] 3 All ER 289; [1998] 2 FLR 550; [1998] 2 FCR 501; 44 BMLR 1; [1998] Fam Law 592; (1998) NLJR 1014; (1998) 29 LS Gaz 27; 142 Sol Jo 195, CA.

R v Collins and Ashworth Hospital Authority ex.p. Brady [2000] Lloyd's Rep Med 335; 58 BMLR 173.

R v Cox 1992, 12 BMLR 38

R v HFEA ex.p. Blood [1997] 2 WLR 807; [1997] 2 All ER 687; [1997] 2 FLR 742; [1997] 2 FCR 501; 35 BMLR 1; [1997] Fam Law 401; (1997) NLJR 253, CA.

R v Salford HA ex.p. Janaway [1989] AC 537; [1988] 3 WLR 1350; [1988] 3 All ER 1079; [1989] 1 FLR 155; (1989) 3 LS Gaz 42; 132 Sol Jo 1731, HL.

R v Smith [1973] 1 WLR 1510; [1974] 1 All ER 376, CA.

R (Pretty) v DPP—see *Pretty v United Kingdom.*

R (Quintavalle) v HFEA—see *Quintavalle v HFEA.*

Rees v UK (1986) 9 EHRR 56; [1987] 2 FLR 111; [1987] Fam Law 157, ECHR.

Robinson v Post Office [1974] 1 WLR 1176; [1974] 2 All ER 737; 117 Sol Jo 915, CA.

Rogers v Whittaker [1993] 4 Med LR 79; (1992) 175 CLR 479; (1992) 109 ALR 625, HC (Aus).

Royal College of Nursing of the United Kingdom v DHSS [1982] AC 800; [1981] 2 WLR 279; [1981] 1 All ER 545; [1981] Crim LR 322; 125 Sol Jo 149, HL.

Salih v Enfield AHA [1991] 3 All ER 400; [1991] 2 Med LR 235; 7 BMLR 1.

Sidaway v. Governors of Bethlem Royal Hospital [1985] AC 871; [1985] 2 WLR 480; [1985] 1 All ER 643; (1985) LS Gaz 1256; (1985) NLJR 203; 129 Sol Jo 154, HL.

Sindicato de Medicos de Asistencia Publica (SIMAP) v Conselleria de Sanidad y Consumo del a Generalidad Valenciana (C303/98) [2001] All ER (EC) 609; [2000] IRLR 845, ECHR.

Skinner v Secretary of State for Transport, The Times 3 January 1995.

Spring v Guardian Assurance [1995] 2 AC 296; [1994] 3 WLR 354; [1994] 3 All ER 129; [1994] IRLR 460; (1994) 40 LS Gaz 36; (1994) NLJR 971; 138 Sol Jo 183, HL.

St George's Healthcare NHS Trust v S; R v Collins ex.p. S [1998] 3 WLR 936; [1998] 3 All ER 673; [1998] 2 FLR 728; [1998] 2 FCR 685; 44 BMLR 160; [1998] Fam Law 526; (1998) 22 LS Gaz 29; (1998) NLJR 693; 142 Sol Jo 164, CA.

T (Consent to Medical Treatment) (Adult Patient), Re: sub nom *T (Adult: Refusal of Treatment), Re:* [1993] Fam 95; [1992] 3 WLR 782; [1992] 2 FLR 458; [1992] 2 FCR 861; [1992] 3 Med LR 306; [1993] Fam Law 27; (1992) NLJR 1125, CA.

Re W (A Minor)(Medical Treatment: Court's Jurisdiction)—see *Re: J (A Minor) (Consent to Medical Treatment).*

W v UK (A/121) (1988) 10 EHRR 29, ECHR.

Whitehouse v Jordan [1981] 1 WLR 246; [1981] 1 All ER 267; 125 Sol Jo 167, HL.

Wieland v Cyril Lord Carpets [1969] 3 All ER 1006.

Wilsher v Essex HA [1988] AC 1074; [1988] 2 WLR 557; [1988] 1 All ER 871; (1988) NLJR 78; 132 Sol Jo 418 & 910, HL.

X *(Minors) v. Bedfordshire County Council* [1995] 2 AC 633; [1995] 3 WLR 152; [1995] 3 All ER 353; [1995] 2 FLR 276; [1995] 3 FCR 337; [1995] Fam Law 537; 94 LS Gaz 313; (1995) NLJR 993, HL.

Appendix 5

Statutes

Abortion Act 1967
Access to Health Records Act 1990
Access to Medical Reports Act 1988
Adults with Incapacity (Scotland) Act 2000
AIDS (Control) Act 1987
Congenital Disabilities Act 1976
Data Protection Act 1998
Freedom of Information Act 2000
Health Act 1999
Health Authorities Act 1995
Health and Social Care Act 2001
Human Fertilization and Embryology Act 1990
Human Rights Act 1998
Medical Act 1983
Medical (Professional Performance) Act 1995
Mental Health Act 1983
Mental Health (Care and Treatment) (Scotland) Act 2003
Mental Health (Patients in the Community) Act 1995
National Health Service and Community Care Act 1990
National Health Service (Primary Care) Act 1997
National Health Service Reform and Health Care Professions Act 2002
National Health Service (Scotland) Act 1978
Offences Against the Person Act 1861
Public Health (Control of Diseases) Act 1984

Directives

Directive 95/46/EC on the protection of individuals in the European Union with regard to the processing of personal data and on the free movement of such data. It took effect from 24 October 1995.

Directive 93/104/EC on the protection of the health and safety of workers in the European Union. It lays down minimum requirements in relation to working hours, rest periods, annual leave and working arrangements for night workers. The Directive was enacted in UK law as the Working Time Regulations, which took effect from 1 October 1998.

Directive 2001/20/EC of the European Parliament and of the Council on the approximation of the laws, regulations and administrative provisions of the Member State relating to the implementation of good clinical practice in the conduct of clinical trials on medicinal products for human use. Official Eur communities 2001;L121:34–44. This is available at: *http://europa.eu.int/eur-lex/pri/en/oj/dat/2001/l_121/l_12120010501en00340044.pdf*

Index

Entries in **bold** indicate tables and entries in *italic* indicate figures

abortion, 17, 18, 42, 89–98, 99–108
  American Supreme Court decisions, **100**, 100
  conscientious objection, 20, 22, 91–2, **92**, 99, 105–7
  emotional trauma, 100
  grounds, 101, **102**
  in Northern Ireland, 97, 99
  partial birth, 92, 93
  religious attitudes, 11, 12, 103–5, **103**
  safety issues, 101–2
  selective, 92
  UK case law, 93–4
Abortion Act (1967), 17, 89, 90–1, **91**, 96, 97
  conscientious objection, 91, **92**, 93
Access to Health Records Act (1990), 39, 42, 44
Access to Medical Reports Act (1988), 39, 41, 44
access to treatment, 18, 22
accountability, 150–1
actus res, 16, 49, 120
Adoption Act (1976), 114
Adults with Incapacity (Scotland) Act (2000), 26, 36–7, 79–85, **80**, 134
  Code of Practice, 84
  continuing powers of attorney, 81–2
  definition of incapacity, 80–1
  glossary of terms, **85**
  intervention/guardianship orders, 83–4
  medical treatment, 82–3
  welfare powers of attorney, 82, 83
advance statements, 37–8, 77, 133
adverse medical events, 149, **150**
advocacy, 74, 75
AIDS (Control) Act (1987), 43
Alder Hey inquiry, 144, **145**
alternative dispute resolution (ADR), 161, 162
altruism, 13
anorexia nervosa, 28, 30, **70**, 70
appraisal, 151, 154
artificial insemination, 109
asbestos exposure, 56–7
assault, 58
assisted suicide, 119, 121–5, 127, **128**
autonomy, 4–5, 8, 14

Bahaism, 105
battery, 58

beneficence, 14
'best interests' of patient, 4, 37–8, 116, 128, 129
bioethics, 8
Bland case, **119**, 119, 120–1, 126–8
Blood case, **111**
blood transfusion, 18, 20, **35**
Bolam case/*Bolam* test, 17, **54**, 54, 128
Bolitho case, 54–5, **55**
brain-stem death, 116–17, **117**
  organ donation, 118
Bristol Inquiry, 150, **151**
Buddhism, 104–5
bullying, **182**, 182

Caesarean section, 18, 26, **32**, 32, 95
Caldicott Report (1997), 43
cardiopulmonary resuscitation (CPR), 132–4
Case Management Conferences (CMC), 161–2
casuistry (case-based reasoning), 13, 14
cervical smear tests, 56
child protection, 50
children
  cardiopulmonary resuscitation (CPR) decision-making, 134
  consent to treatment, 27, 28, 29–31, **30**, **31**
Children Act (1989), 31
Christianity, **8**, 8–10, **10**, 103–4
civil law, 16, **17**
Civil Procedure Rules, 161, 162
civil proceedings, 160–2
  glossary of terms, 163
clinical audit, 152
clinical governance, 152
clinical risk-management, **152**, 152
clinical trials, **139**, 139
Clunis case, 66, **67**
Commission for Health Care Audit and Inspection (CHAI), 153
Commission for Health Improvement (CHI), 153
Commission for Patient and Public Involvement in Health (CPPIH), 153–4
Committee on Professional Performance (CPP), **175**, 175
common law, 16–17
communitarian bioethics, 13, 14
compensation, 16, 19

complaints, 149, 151, **155**, 155, 158, 171
 conciliation, 160
 General Medical Council (GMC) procedures,
  171–2, 173
 written responses, 159
complications of treatment and consent, 25, **33**,
  33–5, 59
compulsory admissions, 19, 68–70
 consent to treatment, 72, 73
 Scottish legislation, **76**, 76–7
compulsory treatment, 19, 65, 66, 72–3
 Scottish legislation, 76–7
conciliation, 160
confidentiality, 39–46, **39**, 42, 159
 Caldicott Report (1997), 43
 disclosure of information, 40–3, **42**
 research data, 139
Congenital Disabilities (Civil Liability) Act (1976),
  52, 96
conscientious objections, 179
 to abortion, 91–2, **92**, 93, 105–7, **180**
consent, 12, 25–38
 applications to court, 29, 36
 children, 20, 27, 28, 29–31
 disclosure of information, **33**, 33, 40
  GMC guidelines, 33–5
 freedom from coercion, 35
 implied, 26–7
 'informed', 35
 life-saving treatment, **35**, 35–6
 mental capacity, 26, 27–8, **31**, 31–2
 mentally disordered patients, 27, 28, 71, 72–3
 negligence claims, **26**, 26, 53, **58**, 58–60
 proxy decision-making, 26
 'prudent patient test', 35
 purposes, 25–6
 refusal, **26**, 26
 removed tissues/organs use, 144–5
 research participation, 27, 139, 140
 review, 27
 screening tests, 27
 stored embryos use, **112**, 112
 validity criteria, 26, 31–6
 written, 26
continuing powers of attorney, 81–2
 see also enduring powers of attorney
continuing professional development (CPD), 151,
  154
Coroner's Inquest, 164, **165**, 166, **168**
 proceedings, 166–8
 verdict, 167
coroner's procedures, 164–8, **168**, **169**
 historical aspects, 164, **165**
 post mortem examinations, 166
 reporting deaths, 164–6, **165**
 statutory duties, 166

Council for the Regulation of Health Care
  Professionals, 155, 157
court procedures, 158–63
 civil proceedings, 160–2
 oral evidence, 160
 preparing evidence, 158–9
Court of Protection, 73
cremation, 10, 11, 12
criminal law, 16, **17**
criminal negligence, 49

Data Protection Act (1998), 39, 41, 42, **44**, 44–5, **45**,
  183
death/dying, 116–25, 126–36
 cardiopulmonary resuscitation (CPR), 132–4
 definitions, 116–18
 disclosure of personal information, 42
 ommision/non-provision of treatment, 119–20,
  126–7
 palliative care, 131
 religious customs, 9–11, 12
 reporting to Coroner, 164–6, **165**
 withdrawal of treatment, 129–30
Deceased Fathers Act (2003), **111**
declaratory relief, 17–18, 36
delayed diagnosis/treatment, 19
deontological theories, 8, 9
designer babies, 113–14, **114**
disciplinary procedures for general practitioners,
  154–5
disclosure of personal information, **33**, 33, 40
 consent, 40–3
 prevention of harm, 41
 sexually transmitted disease, 43
 statutory requirements, 42–3
disproportionate treatment, 14, 129
Do Not Resuscitate (DNR) orders, 18, 132, 134–5, **135**
doctor–patient relationship, 5–6, 9, 35, 39, 179
doctors' professional duties, 156
double/dual effect principle, 123, **131**, 131–2, **132**
driving against medical advice, 41, **42**
duty of care, 47, 49–50, 84, 120
 demonstration of breach, 53–4, **54**
 establishment, 53
 public policy considerations, **50**, 50–1, 57

egg donation, 111, **112**
electroconvulsive therapy (ECT), 28
embryo donation, 109
embryos, 109
 licences for research, **113**, 113
 research (therapeutic) cloning, **144**, 144
 use of stored, **112**, 112
 see also foetus
employers' liability, **51**, 51
employment references, 183

employment rights, **180**, 180
enduring powers of attorney, 36
  see also continuing powers of attorney
Enduring Powers of Attorney Act (1985), 36
ethical theories, 7–8
European Union Clinical Trials directive, 141
European Working Time Directive, 180–1, **181**
euthanasia, 9, 11, 119, 126
  voluntary, 127
experimental treatment, 19

Family Health Services Appeal Authority (FHSAA),
  155
Family Law Reform Act (1969), 30
Fatal Accidents Act (1976), 52
fatherhood, **110**, 110
fees, 7
female cicumcision, 29
fiduciary duty, 84
foetus
  presumed age of viability, 90
  rights/status, 10, 93, 94–5, 115
  use of ovarian tissue, 111, **112**
'four principles' approach (Principlism), 13, 14
Freedom of Information Act (2000), 40
Freeman case, 58

gamete donation, 109, 110–11, **112**
gamete intra-fallopian transfer (GIFT), 109
General Medical Council (GMC), 149, 155–6,
  171–6
  conduct procedures, 173–4
  functions, 171, **172**
  health procedures, 175–6
  letters of advice, 173
  misconduct/deficient performance criteria,
    172–3
  performance procedures, 174–5
  procedures, *173*
Gillick case, **29**, 29–30
Gillick competence, 29, 134
guardianship orders, 71–2, 83
guardianship procedures, 68–70

harassment, 182–3
Health Committee, 175–6
Health and Social Care Act (2001), 45
Helsinki Declaration, 137, 139, **140**, 140–1
Hinduism, **11**, 11–12, 104
Hippocratic oath/Hippocratic tradition, 5–7, **6**, 10,
  39, 126, 179
HIV/AIDS, 43
hormonal implants, 28, 72
hospital orders, 71–2
hospital treatment of offenders, 72
  Scottish legislation, 77

Human Fertilization and Embryology Act (1990), 89,
  92, 93, 98, 109–11
  conscientious objection, 91, **92**
  definitions, 109–10
Human Fertilization and Embryology Authority, 109,
  111–13
  licences for research, **113**, 113
  licences for treatment, 111–12
Human Organ Transplants Act (1989), 118, 119
Human Rights Act (1998), 17, 18–22, **21**, 39, 41, 45
Human Tissues Act (1961), **118**, 118–19, 145
human tissues/organs, 144–6

illegal treatment, 29
in vitro fertilization, 109
Infant Life Preservation Act (1929), 89, **90**, 90
intervention orders, 83
intra-cytoplasmic sperm injection (ICSI), 109
Islam, **10**, 10–11, 104

Judaism, **11**, 11
justice, 14

leave of absence from hopsital, 70
life-saving treatment, 18, **35**, 35–6
Local Medical Committee (LMC), 155
Local Research Ethics Committees (LREC), 141–2

malpractice, 48
Martinez case, 100, *101*
Maynard case, **54**, 54
Medical Register, 155, 156
medical reports, 158–9, **159**
medical school admissions, 107
mens rea, 16, 49, 120, 126, 127
mental capacity, 26, 27–8
  C test, 32
  cardiopulmonary resuscitation (CPR) decision-
    making, 134
  consent, **31**, 31–2
  Mental Health Act Code of Practice (1990), **32**,
    32
  Scottish legislation *see* Adults with Incapacity
    (Scotland) Act (2000)
mental disorder, 27, 28, **68**, 68
  Scottish legislation, 76, 81
mental health, 19, 65–78, **66**
  aftercare, 70–1
  proposed legislation, **67**
Mental Health Act (1983), 28, 65–74, **68**
  admission for treatment, 70
  compulsory admission/guardianship procedures,
    68–70
  consent to treatment, 72–3
  definitions, 68
  glossary of terms, **74**

management of property/affairs of patient, 73
Mental Health Tribunals, 72
  offences, 73–4
  role of courts, 71
Mental Health Act Code of Practice (1990), **32**, 32
Mental Health Care and Treatment (Scotland) Act
    (2003), 65, 74–8, **75**
  glossary of terms, **78**
  rights of users/carers, 77
Mental Health Commission, 73, 80
Mental Health (Patients in the Community) Act
    (1995), **71**, 71
Mental Health Tribunal of Scotland, 75, 77
Mental Health Tribunals, 69, 71, 72
Mental Incapacity Bill, 25, 79, 130
Mental Welfare Commission, 75, 80, 81, 83
methodology (ethical methodology), 13–15
Millan Committee, 74–5
misjudgement, 48
morning-after pill, 92, 96
motherhood, 109–10
Multi-centre Research Ethics Committees (MREC),
    141–2

National Clinical Assessment Authority (NCAA), 155
National Health Service Reform and Health Care
    Professions Act (2002), 153, 155, 157
National Institute for Clinical Excellence (NICE), 153
National Patient Safety Agency (NPSA), 153
National Service Frameworks (NSF), 152
necessity principle, 26, **28**, 28, 72
negligence, **17**, 17, 18, 47–61, **48**, 164
  civil proceedings, 160–2
  claimants, **52**, 52
  congenital disabilities, 96
  contributory, 53
  criminal, 49
  custom test, 51
  defective/inadequate consent, **26**, 26, 53, **58**, 58–60
  defences against liability, **52**, 52–3
  determination of claim, **53**, 53–4
  duty of care, 47, 49–50
  eggshell skull rule, 56
  emotional injury, 100
  establishemnt of causality ('but for' test), 55–6, **56**
    intervening acts, 55, **57**, 57
  inexperienced doctors, **57**–8
  limitation period, 52
  NHS Indemnity, 51–2
  proximity/foreseeability of harm, 56–7
  public policy considerations, **50**, 50–1, 57
  terminology, 48
  vicarious liability, 51
neurosurgery, 28–9, 72, 77
NHS Indemnity, 51–2
non-maleficience, 14

Northern Ireland abortion law, 97, 99
notifiable communicable diseases, 41, **42**, 42
novus actus interveniens, 55, 57
Nuremberg Code, 137, **138**, 139, 141
Nuremberg Doctors' Trial, 137–8, **138**, 141

Offences Against the Person Act (1861), 89–90, **90**,
    96, 97, 99
oral evidence, 160
organ donation, 10, 11, 12, 28, 118
organizational standards, 151–2

palliative care, 14, 131
parental orders, 110–11
partial birth abortion, 92, 93
Patients' forums, 153
Perruche case, **97**
persistent vegetative state, **117**, 117–18, 119, 120,
    126–9
  Practice Note of Official Solicitor, **121–2**, 121
personality disorder, 65, 66
Police and Criminal Evidence Act (1984), 43
post mortem examination, 10, 11, 12
  coroner's procedures, 166
  use of retained tissues/organs, 145
post-modern ethics, 13, 15
postcode prescribing, 18, 19, 22
posthumous conception, **111**
pre-implantation genetic analysis, 113–14, **114**
Preliminary Proceedings Committee (PPC), 172,
    173–4
Pretty case, 121, **122**, 122–3
Principlism ('four principles' approach), 13, 14
Procurator Fiscal, 164, 168–70, **169**
Professional Conduct Committee (PCC), 174, **175**
professional regulation, 149–57, **151**
proportionate treatment, 129
Protection from Harassment Act (1997), 182
proxy decision-making, 25, 26, 27, 36, 79, 83, 116,
    134
psychopathic disorder, 70, 71
Public Guardian, 79, 80, 81

rashness, 48
rationing of healthcare, 19
reason, 5
recklessness, 48, 49
refusal of treatment, 26, 26, 32, 35
  advance statements, 37
  Caesarean section, 18, 26, **32**, 32, 95
  children, 30, 31
  life-saving treatment, 35, 36
  mental health legislation, 65, 66
relentless therapy *see* disproportionate treatment
religious beliefs/attitudes, **7**, 7–9, **8**, 20, 103–5, **103**
remand for report on mental condition, 71

remand for treatment, 71, 77
removal to place of safety, 69–70
reproductive technology, 109–15, **110**
res ipsa loquitur, 55
research, 137–46
    Adults with Incapacity (Scotland) Act (2000), 83
    assisted reproduction, **113**, 113
    beneficience, 139, 140–1
    confidentiality of information, 139
    consent, 27, 139, 140
    on embryos (research/therapeutic cloning), **144**, 144
    justice, 139, 141
    respect for persons, 139, 140
    safety issues, 139, 140–1
    use of human tissues/organs, 144–6
Research Ethics Committees, 141–4
    ethical review process, **143–4**, 143–4
    membership requirements, 142
    remit, 142
    working procedures, 142–3
research (therapeutic) cloning, **144**, 144
restriction order, 72
retrolental fibroplasia, **56**, 56
revalidation, 154, 156
right to life, 18, 106–7
rights of doctors, 179–83, **180**
Rogers v *Whittaker*, **59**, 59

Scottish Mental Health Care and Treatment Act
    (2003), 65, 74–8
screening tests, 27
selective abortion, 92
sex selection, 113–14, **114**
sexually transmitted disease, 43
Sheriff Court, 81
Shipman case, 124–5
Sidaway case, **33**, 33, **59**, 59
Sikhism, **11**, 11–12, 105
social justice, 5

standard of proof, 16, 49
standards of care, 19
statute law, 16–17
Statutory Instruments, 16, 17
sterilization, 17–18, 27–8, 29
suicide, 9, 11
    assisted/physician-assisted, 119, 121–5, 127, **128**
supervised discharge, **67**, 71
surrogacy, 109, 114
Surrogacy Arrangements Act (1985), 114

terminology, 4–5
therapeutic (research) cloning, **144**, 144
trolley waits in A&E, 19
trust, 5, 6, 179–80

unconscious patient, 34
utilitarianism, 12–13

vicarious liability, 51
virtue ethics, 13
voluntary euthanasia, 127

welfare powers of attorney, 82, 83
whistle-blowing, 181–2
Wilsher case, **56**, 56, 58
withdrawal of hydration and nutrition, 17, 18, 119,
    120–1, 126–9
    dying patient, 130
    non-dying patient, 130
    Practice Note of Official Solicitor, **121–2**, 121
withdrawal of ventilation, 123
withdrawal/withholding of treatment, 129–30, **135**,
    135–6
    conscientious objection, 130–1
    GMC guidance, 130
witness statements, 158, **159**
wrongful birth, 96, 97, 106–7
wrongful conception/pregnancy, 96
wrongful life, 96–7, **97**, 106–7

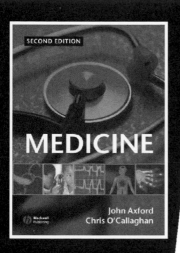

Medicine
Second Edition

John S Axford and Christopher A O'Callaghan

Published April 2004
1248 pages 872 illustrations
ISBN **0632051620** Paperback

- **Focused on the core curriculum**

- **Clinically orientated throughout**

- **No unnecessary detail**

- **Highly-structured for easy learning & revision**

- **Exactly the right level of detail for every topic**

- **Comprehensively visual to aid the learning process**

- **Value for money**

Medicine is a revolutionary core textbook designed with students for students.

The book successfully integrates basic science and clinical practice. The systems-based chapters all follow a common structure:

- **Structure and Function** - the essential basics that underpin each system

- **Approach to the Patient** - history and examination, clinical presentations, differential diagnosis and investigations

- **Disease and their Management** - all the common conditions that medical students need to know for future practice

This consistent, easy-to-navigate structure makes locating information simple and it is also tailored toward successful revision. All chapters have been updated, with colour-coded features.

Revised to follow the core curriculum and current medical practice.

For more details information on this fantastic brand new text, log onto

Blackwell
Publishing

www.blackwellpublishing.com/axford

Medical Statistics at a Glance

First Edition

Aviva Petrie and Caroline Sabin
June 2000. 144 pages 124 illustrations
ISBN 0632050756 Paperback £15.95

*Worked examples to accompany each topic

*Emphasis on computer analysis of data rather than hand calculations

*Supported by a website at www.medstatsaag.com - this site contains useful self-assessment questions to aid student learning

In line with the other books in the At a Glance series, this new addition leads the reader through a number of self-contained topics, each covering a different aspect of medical statistics. The majority of these use the standard 'At a Glance' format of two pages per topic.

The authors have provided a basic introduction to the underlying concepts of medical statistics and a guide to the most commonly used statistical procedures. Topics describing a statistical technique are accompanied by a worked example, using real data, illustrating its use. Where possible, the same data set has been used in more than one topic to reflect the reality of data analysis. Detailed and complex hand calculations have been avoided with a concentration on the interpretation of computer data analysis.

Medical Statistics at a Glance is versatile in its use as an explanation, a revision summary and a long-term source of reference.

Blackwell
Publishing

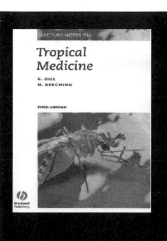

Lecture Notes on Tropical Medicine

Fifth Edition

Geoff Gill and Nick Beeching
February 2004. 368 pages 86 illustrations
ISBN 063206496X Paperback £16.95

- **Emphasis on the clinical aspects of problem solving and management in the tropics**

- **Emphasises a problem-based clinical approach using clinical presentations**

- **An increased global approach to medicine in the tropics not just tropical and exotic diseases**

Lecture Notes on Tropical Medicine is a core text with an emphasis on the practical aspects of problem-solving in the tropics. It is a very practical companion for the increasing number of medical students and junior doctors who have the opportunity to practice medicine in the tropics.

This new, revised edition includes a more global and syndromic approach to tropical medicine. In addition to covering the serious and relevant tropical diseases, the book also covers conditions and diseases that are becoming more widespread in the tropics such as epilepsy, diabetes and AIDS.

Carefully selected colour plates and an increased number of illustrations, effectively portray clinical conditions. This edition includes a separate section on HIV and reflects the impact that AIDS has had on the tropics.

- New chapter on non-communicable diseases, such as epilepsy, diabetes and heart disease, which are becoming more wide spread in the tropics

- New chapter on refugee health that covers humanitarian disasters, control of epidemics and health assessment of asylum seekers

- Over 25 expert contributors

For more details information or to order your copy, log onto

www.blackwellmedstudent.com

Blackwell
Publishing

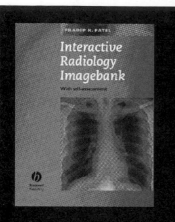

Interactive Radiology Imagebank

Pradip R Patel
February 2004
ISBN 1405101040 CD £19.95

From Pradip Patel, the best selling author of Lecture Notes on Radiology a complete learning reference and self-test resource.

This easy-to-install CD-ROM contains a comprehensive databank of Radiology Images and Self-Assessment material.

The collection includes 1000 Radiology Images, 400 Radiological Case Histories, 200 Multiple Choice Questions and a selection of video clips of key radiological procedures.

This CD-ROM has been designed for use by anyone wanting to improve their skills in radiological diagnosis, in particular clinical medical students, junior doctors and trainee radiographers. It can also be used in conjunction with Lecture Notes on Radiology, to supplement and reinforce learning.

* for use both as a stand-alone or companion to Lecture Notes on Radiology

* a great tool for honing and testing clinical diagnostic skills

* easy to install; up and running in minutes

* 1,000 radiological images

* 400 case histories test the users diagnostic thinking

* 200 MCQs for use prior to a clinical exam. Users can choose to test themselves at basic, intermediate or advanced level

* video clips show details of actual clinical procedurestributors

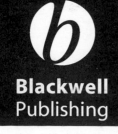

Blackwell
Publishing